# The Life That Lives on Man

# The Life That Lives on Man

## Michael Andrews

Arrow Books

Arrow Books Limited
17-21 Conway Street, London W1P 6JD

An imprint of the Hutchinson Publishing Group

London Melbourne Sydney Auckland
Johannesburg and agencies
throughout the world

First published by Faber & Faber Ltd 1976
Arrow edition 1978
Reprinted 1984

© Michael L. A. Andrews 1976

Printed and bound in Great Britain by
Anchor Brendon Ltd, Tiptree, Essex

ISBN 0 09 916500 7

# **Contents**

# Illustrations

# 1
# Attitudes

When the murdered body of Thomas à Becket lay cooling on the
flags of Canterbury Cathedral his attendants, removing the linen
covering to his penitential hair shirt, burst into alternate weeping
and laughter to see his garment 'seethe like a simmery cauldron'
with lice. The courtiers of Peter the Great were chronicled as
parading through the streets of London indiscriminately dropping pearls and lice; and Pepys wrote in his *Diary* that he had to
return a new periwig to his barber to have it cleaned of nits,
'which vexed me cruelly that he should put such a thing into my
hands'.

Parasites were an accepted accompaniment to life, though it
did not do to draw attention to them. In seventeenth-century
France it was considered most improper to take lice or fleas or
other vermin and crack them between one's finger-nails in
company 'except in the most intimate circles', and George
Washington when he was fourteen copied out 'Rules of Civility'
including the commandment 'Kill no vermin, as fleas, lice, ticks,
etc. in the sight of others.' The story goes that one of Louis XI's
courtiers removed a flea from the King's lace and was suitably
rewarded with gold, but when another over-avaricious colleague
repeated the same action the next day the irate King had him
whipped.

To most people the very suggestion that they might be
infested with vermin is utterly repulsive, not even mentionable.
We associate such insects with the black squalor of the Middle
Ages, with periods of decadence when clothes were never
changed, and with *coiffures* so extravagant and uncombable that
they were even nested in by mice. But while we are socially blind
to our parasites we are in the midst of an epidemic.

*The Life That Lives on Man*

The human flea has almost disappeared, true enough, sucked out of existence by the vacuum cleaner. But the unswept 5 centimetres of fitted carpet round the skirting have become a centrally heated preserve for the cat flea which now bites us instead.

Florence Nightingale steadfastly refused to believe in bacteria, but they still killed her patients. Most mothers and not a few local authorities now refuse to contemplate the head louse, but in 1970 a survey of Teesside school children revealed that 15 per cent of the children were literally lousy. The percentage was as high as 26·5 in some secondary schools and a responsible estimate put the number of infested heads in Britain at one and a half million. A revolting and unrecognized public health problem was revealed, all the more sinister for the knowledge that the head louse is resistant to DDT and can be the means of spreading typhus, one of the deadliest of man's diseases. Although lice are transmitted quickly from child to child the source of an infestation that cannot be cleaned up is almost always the parents.

The insect plague is by no means confined to the dirty and underprivileged; lice are as happy on clean hair as on dirty, as partial to blue blood as to red. The parasites of the human body have no respect for social frontiers, and while the current pandemic of VD has been sweeping the Western World there has been a rapid rise in the number of cases of crab lice. One celebrated lady entomologist told me with relish that she had observed crab lice in the eyelashes of one of Her Britannic Majesty's Ambassadors, though she declined to tell me which one. Since crabs are usually transmitted during sexual contact and move directly from hair to hair, the observation throws an interesting light on the amatory attitudes of His Excellency.

If a hasty survey in the mirror leaves you crab-free, look at your face a little more closely with a high-powered magnifying glass, and you may well glimpse the tail of the mite *Demodex* retreating into the follicle of one of your eyelashes. Some authorities believe that all of us harbour this beast in the warm oily fastnesses of our sebaceous glands; though for something

10

which lives under their very noses it is remarkably little studied, and nobody knows exactly what it does. If this search is unrewarded try scraping a little of the dust from under one of the buttons of your mattress and look at it under a low-powered microscope. The chances are that you will find it well populated with the dust mite patiently devouring the flakes of your shed skin which drop through the sheets. And that black dust which seems to be everywhere in the Underground in London? That is skin too, shed by a generation of strap-hangers. Each tiny flake supports its own population of bacteria which float in a thin haze through the air before being inhaled to colonize another lung.

The horrid truth is that each of us has about as many bacteria and yeasts on the surface of his or her skin as there are people on earth; far from being 'clean' after a bath the number of organisms released from the surface actually goes up as they emerge from the nooks and skinny crannies where they multiply. It is time to take a new look at the back of our hands and to realize that our skins are a habitat which supports a whole flora and fauna of creatures which have evolved with us through millennia. However hard we may wish to retreat from our animal origins we will not be able to escape our fellow travellers. The huge majority, numerically, are harmless or beneficial. But then the huge majority are also invisible and earn our indifference. It is the secretive hopping and creeping progress of larger creatures which brings the shudders, but insects are only the most conspicuous as well as the most infrequent inhabitants of our own private zoological gardens.

If by now you are scratching it is an instinctive and helpful reaction to the presence of parasites, but we are so unused to considering our true nature that the knowledge of just what is bugging you may leave you uncomfortable and even sleepless.

Bacteriologists are usually regarded by their hospital colleagues as having an obsessive regard for the trifling – again, a remarkable denial of their close aquaintance with the germs which ultimately govern our life or death. But they themselves forget how little we are aware of the world they study. One bacteriologist, Theodor Rosebury, once made the mistake of taking a sample of tartar from the teeth of a charlady with infected gums. Inadvisedly he allowed her to take first look down the microscope in front of a class of medical students. The next time he saw her she had had all her teeth out.

To put in perspective our fastidious denial of our real nature, it is worth while to note how the discovery of minute organisms affected their contemporary observers. The Dutchman Anton van Leeuwenhoek (pronounced Laywenhook) developed a remarkable skill in making tiny lenses through which he made the first truly scientific observations of life in miniature in the mid-seventeenth century. His letters to the Royal Society provoked the wonder of the world. His house soon became an attraction for gentlefolk visiting Delft, and he nicely records the paradox of their interest.

I have had several gentlewomen in my house, who were keen on seeing the little eels in vinegar [*nematodes*]; but some of them were so disgusted at the spectacle that they vowed they'd never use vinegar again. But what if one should tell such people in future that there are more animals living in the scum on the teeth in a man's mouth, than there are men in a whole kingdom?

The fascination of the minute, and the discovery of the unpleasant reality beneath the illusion of human beauty were soon seized by contemporary writers. Jonathan Swift made the most explicit use of the world in miniature when he allowed Gulliver to be inspected by the keen eyes of the Lilliputians.

I took him up in my hand and brought him close; which he confessed was at first a very shocking sight. He said he could discover great holes in my skin; that the stumps of my beard were ten times stronger than the bristles of a boar; and my complexion made up of several colours altogether disagreeable.

On a later voyage he encounters Brobdingnagian lice:

I could see distinctly the limbs of these vermin with my naked eye, much better than those of a European louse through the microscope; and their snouts with which they rooted like swine.

Following the scientific fervour of the times he wishes to dissect one 'although indeed the sight was so nauseous that it perfectly turned my stomach'.

Though Leeuwenhoek discovered bacteria it was not until two centuries had elapsed that Pasteur related their presence to disease. His reward was a morbid fear of dirt and infection. Pasteur even avoided shaking hands for fear of a chance contamination, and one of his assistants records how he carefully wiped his plate and glass before dining.

He minutely inspected the bread that was served to him and placed on the table-cloth everything he found in it: small fragments of wool, of roaches, of flour worms.

With an air of regret he goes on:

Often I tried to find in my own piece of bread from the same loaf the objects found by Pasteur but could not discover anything.

If, in a nineteenth-century world of drains and disinfectant, cleanliness was next to godliness, in our own generation the slaughter of germs became a religion, evangelized nightly on the television at a cost rivalling that of building cathedrals. But suddenly it has begun to dawn on the human consciousness that the presence of germs on skin might not be something wholly undesirable. Suddenly the conquest of BO and all the other anti-social smells which, if you are persuaded by the millions of pounds spent on promoting the idea, assault the nostrils of your neighbours, became not only wrong but positively harmful. With the knowledge of the finite nature of our earth and the interdependence of all its inhabitants came the popular appreciation of ecology. Just as the wholesale use of DDT and Dieldrin came to be abhorred for their disruption of fragile natural systems of life in the wild, so the intimate deodorant spray was discovered to pose not just a threat of frostbite to the private parts, but also to decimate the natural populations of bacteria which held their evil cousins at bay.

There are over two million species of animals and plants. We are just one of those species, at the mercy of the smallest virus or bacterium. Yet knowing our place within the life that lives upon us gives us the vision of a strange new world, beautiful in its complexity and wonderful in its precision.

> Pull down thy vanity, it is not man
> Made courage, or made order, or made grace,
>    Pull down thy vanity, I say pull down.
> Learn of the green world what can be thy place
> In scaled invention or true artistry,
> Pull down thy vanity . . .
> The green casque has outdone your elegance.
>
> EZRA POUND *(from* Canto LXXXI)

# 2
# Exploration of the World in Miniature

It is hard to imagine ourselves living in a world where there was no scientific explanation for disease. Bad air, damps, the stars, the elements, the evil eye, the humours, the wind, almost everything susceptible to man's five senses was blamed for contagion. It was only natural to suspect the known rather than the unknown. So the conditions which caused the spread of infection were often blamed rather than the agent of infection itself. Sometimes by the most remarkable coincidence the right preventive measures were discovered. When it was universally believed that malaria was caused by bad air from the swamps, some unrecorded genius discovered that a fine wire mesh put in windows would keep the pestilential miasma away. The fact that malaria is carried not by bad air but by the anopheles mosquito made no difference to the beneficial result. Draining swamps also reduced the disease. What could be more natural than to deduce that swampy air was infective?

It is not surprising then, that tradition has it that the first disease whose cause was established beyond doubt was scabies, the itch. The scabies mite is just visible to the naked eye and has been known longer than history. Epicurus was impressed by its small size and maintained that it was not made of atoms but was an atom itself. And Shakespeare acknowledges its presence, and even its cure, when Mercutio describes Queen Mab's chariot on the way to the Capulets' ball in *Romeo and Juliet*.

> Her waggoner, a small grey-coated gnat,
> Not half so big as a round little worm
> Pricked from the lazy finger of a maid.

Today the incidence of the 'round little worm' and its power of spreading can be judged from the fact reported by a British doctor working in the refugee camps that 50 per cent of the refugees from East Bengal who fled to India at the time of the Bangladesh war had scabies. Ironically, as detailed in a later chapter, most general practitioners in the West fail to recognize the symptoms.

It stands to reason that before the discovery of the lens nothing, no process invisible to the naked eye, could be explained without recourse to myth and conjecture. Also the scarcity of books and literacy ensured that the correct observations of one generation were frequently lost to the next. So Homer writing the *Iliad* over seven hundred years before the birth of Christ makes Achilles warn of the danger that flies will slip into the open wounds of Patroklos and there produce maggots. But Ovid at the time of Christ wrote that wasps were spontaneously generated from dead horses while beetles came from the bodies of asses. Pliny, who wrote the *Historia Naturalis* before his scientific curiosity led him to his death in the great eruption of Vesuvius, wrote that some insects 'are engendered by filth, acted upon by the rays of the sun', and that others with wings came from damp dust in corners.

The origin of life was of course primarily a religious question and we find St Augustine wondering how spontaneous generation could be reconciled with the biblical stories of the Creation and the Great Flood. His contemporaries believed that bees came from sweat dropped from the brows of Negro slaves, and one is filled with sympathy for Huxley's complaint that the great tragedy of science is the slaying of a beautiful hypothesis by an ugly fact.

If insects could be made out of nothing, then the opportunities for travellers' tall tales were plentiful. In the fourteenth century Mandeville claims he found a tree whose huge melon-shaped fruit he ate. In it, he wrote, he found a lamb. He described how when the fruit ripened and fell the lamb's legs grew into the ground and it ate only grass within reach. In fact Mandeville never made any journeys and only compiled the writings of others. When science is bedevilled by downright lies it can only proceed when all suspect evidence is eliminated. The legend of the vegetable lamb was not finally laid to rest until, in the eighteenth century, Count von Linné, also known as Linnaeus, systematically examined specimens of all the plants believed to fruit as lambs. Perhaps the hardest task of naturalists has been ridding science of speculation unsupported by observation.

The old confusion between source and cause persisted until the Renaissance and the coming of scientific method. We see Francis Bacon, who did much to promote modern scientific observation, nevertheless describing fleas as being bred principally from straw or mats, and not until the introduction of the lens to Europe at the start of the seventeenth century were Aristotle and Galen superseded as the source of all scientific truth. The lens had been known to the Arabs since the ninth century. It was not so much the unlocking of the secrets of nature which proved the challenge, but the superseding of old beliefs and dogmas.

Just as the lenses of Galileo shattered man's instinctive belief that the sun and heavens revolved around the earth so also they led to a challenging of the philosophy of casual creation, although the final refutation of spontaneous generation did not come until Pasteur and his contemporaries proved that a meat broth would not decompose if it was sealed off from contaminating bacteria. That was little more than a century ago, 250 years after Galileo observed with a lens that insects had compound eyes.

The importance of understanding the life-cycle of insects was chiefly the light it threw on the process of putrefaction. Once decomposing matter had been seen to be a breeding ground and not an independent source of flies and other insects, the way was open to realize the role of contagion and the origins of disease.

As early as 1546 Fracastoro of Verona had held that disease was spread by invisible *semina* or seeds. It is likely that our own use of the word 'germ' is almost as old. The religious philosophers were already beginning to reach the inevitable conclusion from piety, since they felt it impossible that flies on which the

Almighty had expended so much wisdom and art could arise just by chance from refuse. But it was the English physician William Harvey, chiefly known for his discovery of the circulation of the blood, who put the matter into print in 1651 with his book *Omnia ex Ovo* whose frontispiece shows fish, insects, animals, and even man springing from the egg, still however respectably grasped in the hand of almighty Zeus.

Trade, navigation and the study of geography proved the spurs driving forward the interest in science, and it was no accident that the great trading nations of the age, England and Holland, should have the men of wealth and leisure who could devote their time to observations of Nature. The first institution for teaching the new science in England was Gresham College, and it was there that the Royal Society of London for Improving Natural Knowledge first met under patronage of King Charles II in 1662. The concern of the Society with observation rather than speculation was made clear in its second Royal Charter:

> ... whose studies are to be applied to further promoting by the authority of experiments the sciences of natural things and of useful Arts ... to the glory of God the Creator and the advantage of the human race.

Its members paid a shilling a week as subscription, but King Charles not only never paid a penny, but never actually visited a meeting of the Society during his lifetime. He 'mightily laughed' at the notion of men who could devote themselves 'only in weighing of ayre'. Yet as Robert Hooke wrote in his letter to the King at the front of his famous book of microscopical observations, *Micrographia*: 'The calm prosperity of your Reign has given us the leisure to follow these studies of quiet and retirement.'

The new passion for knowledge of the natural world provoked ample scepticism. One publican described the Royal Society's museum as a

> warehouse of Egyptian mummies, old musty skeletons of men, women and monkeys, birds, beasts and fishes; abortives put up in pickle, and an abundance of other memorandums of mortality.

In one respect his contempt for curios was justified, the age of systematic collection and classification had not yet come. The new scientists were to progress by experiment, and it was the dexterity of the craftsman building experimental apparatus which was to bring the results. The greatest of these was Robert Hooke, the son of a poor clergyman in the Isle of Wight. He was employed by the Hon. Robert Boyle, one of the band of brilliant young men to found the Royal Society.

Hooke probably carried out most of Boyle's experiments with gases, and he was soon made curator of experiments. At the age of twenty-nine he published *Micrographia* (1665). Sir Christopher Wren helped him to produce the plates which illustrated this first systematic account of the world seen through the magnifying glass. The same two men were later to collaborate on the plans for the reconstruction of London after the Great Fire, and Hooke is credited with drawing the plans for the Monument, which still commemorates the Fire. Wren's greatest architectural achievement was St Paul's Cathedral. But it is likely that Hooke's work on the stability of arches made from masonry was crucial to the design of St Paul's dome.

Once the intellectual climate became receptive to new knowledge the whole gamut of man's pent-up curiosity was released. While Robert Hooke was making his elegant engravings of the flea and louse, 'a creature so officious that 'twill be known to everyone at one time or another', the Tuscan physician Francesco Redi published the first specially devised experiments on the development of insects from which he concluded that rotting matter was nothing more than a convenient nest for eggs. Later still Leeuwenhoek watched the metamorphosis from egg to larva to chrysalis to flea and concluded: 'Fleas are not produced by corruption, but in the ordinary way of generation.'

It is only by developing more powerful tools that one genius can improve on the detailed observations of another, and the knowledge of our parasites progressed as the tools at our disposal became more and more sophisticated. The process still continues: fleas have even been made radioactive recently so that their movements can be traced in the wild.

Leeuwenhoek had a remarkable ingenuity in grinding lenses – it is said that he once ground a lens from a grain of sand to look at a grain of sand – but he also had that other most essential gift of the naturalist: acute powers of observation. Born in 1632 he was a draper and haberdasher living in the street still called the Hippolytusbuurt in Delft. He was a prosperous man being both a qualified surveyor and appointed as wine-gauger and weights and measures inspector to the town. On one occasion he acted as official receiver of the assets of Jan Vermeer, but his claim to fame lies in his skill in the use of his 'microscopes'. These were not the compound double-lens microscopes which first appeared in Holland about ten years before his birth, but minute single lenses mounted in a metal plate with an arrangement of screw adjustments to bring the specimen into focus on the end of a pin. With these crude but effective instruments Leeuwenhoek became the first man to see bacteria.

Leeuwenhoek did make doublet and triplet combinations of lenses but the power of magnification came from the very short focal length possible with a tiny lens. Possibly because of the difficulty of focusing, or because of their value as curios, Leeuwenhoek apparently kept his specimens permanently mounted on different microscopes which gave a magnification of up to two hundred diameters at a focal length of one-fifth of an inch. Catalogued at his death were 419 such lenses, each with its specimen such as: 'the sting and sheath of a flea, the feet of a flea, and the sting, skin and ovipositor of a louse'.

At that time there were the first stirrings of an international scientific community based on the Royal Society in London, and it was to them that Leeuwenhoek wrote, humbly supplying his observations on mould, the sting and mouthparts of a bee, and on the louse. These were duly published in 1673 in the *Philosophical Transactions*, the journal of the Society. The correspondence continued until his death, the Royal Society variously misspelling his name in eighteen different ways – the Italians even spelt it Le Wenocchio – and he bequeathed to the Royal Society twenty-six silver-mounted microscopes each with its own specimen in a special travelling case. These the Society succeeded in losing, but fortunately not before measurements on the efficacy of the lenses had been made.

Leeuwenhoek's most famous observations were those which led to his discovery of 'little animalcules', now known to be protozoa and bacteria.

In an attempt to find out why pepper was hot to the tongue he put pepper in water to soften it for three weeks. On 24 April 1676 'I saw therein, with great wonder, incredibly many little animalcules, of divers sorts.' He goes on to describe various forms of protozoa:

> The fourth sort of little animal which drifted among the three sorts aforesaid, were incredibly small; nay so small, in my sight, that I judged that even if 100 of these very wee animals lay stretched out one against another, they could not reach to the length of a grain of coarse sand; and if this be true, then ten hundred thousand of these living creatures could scarce equal the bulk of a coarse sand-grain.

He had already defined the size of his coarse sand-grain as a unit of measurement about one-thirtieth of an inch long. On other occasions he used the eye of a louse as another international standard of measurement! Later Leeuwenhoek estimated that there were up to eight million bacteria in a drop of water and drew the sceptical criticism of the Royal Society. However, they repeated his pepper-water experiment with the same results, and even demonstrated the animalcules to King Charles who was 'very well pleased'.

A few months after Leeuwenhoek's letter describing bacteria was published in the *Philosophical Transactions*, a correspondent noted that the

> discoveries are exceeding curious, and may prompt us to suspect that our Air is also vermiculated, and perhaps most of all in long calms, long-lasting Eastern winds, or much moisture in Spring-time, and in seasons of general infection in man and animals.

There was no proof, the letter was forgotten, and the first scientific experiments on transmissible microbial diseases were not to be done for a century and a half.

Leeuwenhoek went on to observe blood, sweat, faeces and urine in search of more of his little animalcules. But he remained fascinated that in spite of daily rubbing his teeth with salt there was always a little white matter left between them. 'I then most always saw, with great wonder, that in the said matter there were many very little living animalcules, very prettily a-moving.' He was interested to find that the number of bacteria was greater in people who had never cleaned their teeth and he also observed that vinegar would kill bacteria – but not if they were safe inside the white matter (tartar) on the teeth. It seems surprising to us that he should not have made the connection between bacteria and putrefaction, but often the greatest discoveries seem the simplest in retrospect.

One of Leeuwenhoek's party tricks was to demonstrate the blood circulation in the tail of an eel using a special apparatus. In 1698 he was honoured to show this capillary blood-flow to Tsar Peter the Great, the founder of St Petersburg and the Russian Navy. Whether his retinue were also showed close-ups of their lice, history does not relate.

Scientific observation was still very much a preserve of the wealthy, practised either by the merchant class such as Leeuwenhoek, or by those enjoying the patronage of the nobility. This was not the most fertile soil for objectivity, and science even today is still not free from the taint of religious and political dogma. Louis XIV's Court Physician Pierre Boral wrote a collection of observations in 1656 in which he praised the wonders revealed by the lens:

> Through which atoms become quasi-visible and minute insects are changed into a colossal monster; with the aid of which countless parts are discovered in these living atoms; and day after day, doors of the new Physics are opened; so much so that God's Majesty becomes more illuminated by these tiny Bodies than in gigantic ones, and their perplexing constitution convinces even the most godless, and leads them

to the notion, the admiration and the veneration of their supreme Maker.

The religious awe seems just a shade too effusive. Certainly the irreligious feelings of the plain man are better represented by Rabbie Burns's famous poem 'To a Louse, on seeing one on a lady's bonnet at church':

> Ye ugly, creepin, blastit wonner,
> Detested, shunn'd, by saunt an' sinner,
> How daur ye set your fit upon her
> Sae fine a Lady!
> Gae somewhere else and seek your dinner,
> On some poor body.

Although that was written over a century later.

Patronage of early scientists by kings led to the unfortunate consequence that their discoveries became the subject of fashion. Woe betide the court microscopist who did not produce wonders to equal those of his neighbouring principality. This led in some cases to a systematic piracy of other work. For example the French microscopist Joblot printed exact facsimiles of Hooke's engravings of cheese mites claiming them as his own. So it is not surprising to find that Leeuwenhoek never revealed the secret of how he made his best observations. He admitted that he had a method which revealed far better detail than holding up his lenses to the light. It now seems almost certain that he had discovered what is now known as dark-ground illumination, where the object is lit whilst the background is in darkness: precisely the illumination which makes motes visible in a shaft of sunlight in a darkened room.

It was perhaps fitting that Leeuwenhoek, who had no equal as a microscopist for 150 years afterwards, should have made the most important of all the observations on the origin of life. One day a medical student noticed movement in the sperm of a man treated for venereal disease and brought it to his attention. Leeuwenhoek later wrote to Henry Oldenburg, the first Secretary of the Royal Society, with apologies for raising a subject which might be thought distasteful, careful to point out that his observations were made from material 'from the overplus of marital intercourse and without committing any sin'. This sperm he found to be 'crowded with an infinity of animals like tadpoles'. He was once again astonished by their number and pointed out that they appeared to exceed the entire population of the earth, for whose presence they could claim responsibility.

The debate on the generation of life was to echo on for centuries but careful scientific observation had already begun to restrict the excesses of the philosophers and to put man into his context in Nature.

# 3

# Our Skin as an Eco-System

*All the wise world is little else, in Nature,*
*But parasites and sub-parasites.*
                                        BEN JONSON

To come to terms with the life on one's skin, one's most intimate companions, it helps to know friend from foe. The flea, which seems no more than a harmless irritant, is through no fault of its own perhaps man's most deadly enemy, while some forms of the bacteria which are usually treated with indiscriminate dread as germs may be precious friends. So it is quite wrong to jumble all together as noxious parasites. Asked to define the role of a parasite one would be forgiven for replying like the tramp, 'Search me!' But in science parasitism has an exact meaning. Strictly the word means one who eats beside another, but the modern usage implies dependence. A parasite is a creature living at the expense of another, derived by sudden chance or millions of tiny evolutionary steps from free-living ancestors. Some, like many of the sucking mosquitoes, bugs and ticks, originally evolved as suckers of the juices of plants. It has even been suggested that the *Plasmodium* causing malaria was first sucked by a mosquito from a plant. These forms of life developed before mammals and birds, but somewhere along the evolutionary path some adventurous individual by accident or design sucked blood instead and found it a superior diet. From being an attractive habit, in the span of a few million generations it became a necessity, and at this point the parasite is caught in an evolutionary trap. Huxley defined biological progress as 'control over environment and independence from it', but the tick or flea which is confined to one mammalian species has its destiny irreversibly bound up with that species. It is too late to find out whether the Dodo had specific parasites in its nest because they too will be extinct.

A well-adapted parasite must obviously not be fatal to its host, or at least not until its host has bred to ensure future meals on its young. So the association of certain human parasites like the flea and louse with fatal diseases is as dangerous for the parasite as it is for man. The mortality of man from plague runs perhaps into hundreds of millions, but the mortality of fleas must have been infinitely greater. Not only is the plague bacillus often fatal to the insect, but without blood meals from its host the insect cannot breed, and the natural host of the plague-flea is the rat, the first animal to succumb to an epidemic.

A parasite is usually recognized as an irritant, and it must also evade the search-and-destroy missions of its host. Many an injudicious flea has ended as a bloody-smear between thumb and finger-nail. So it is not surprising to find that in addition to direct parasitism, other degrees of dependence have arisen. By being more favourable to the host these provide a more secure relationship for the dependant. Commensalism is the harmless association of two animals in which only one derives the benefit. Again the scientific interpretation is not quite the same as the 'table-sharing' derivation means. Seagulls following the plough, the robin perched on the spade, and most of the bacteria living off the secretions of our skin, all gain from our lives without doing us injury. They have our indulgence just so long as they do us no harm.

A further step towards security of tenure has been taken by the animals which have paired with a host in an association which benefits both. The farmyard cat earns its keep by mousing, the cattle egret keeps its host free from ticks. This form of mutual benefit is called symbiosis and it appears in astonishingly diverse forms. The cow yields milk in exchange for shelter and food; but the assassin-bug of Venezuela has a fungus in its intestine which passes from one generation to the next on the surface of the eggshells and in the faeces which are eaten by the nymphs after they hatch. If the young insect is deprived of the fungus it fails to develop normally, and even those few which metamorphose to the adult form are sterile. The fates have inextricably entwined the lives of fungus and bug.

Even stranger to our eyes are the symbiotic relationships of bacteria with some deep-sea fish. Certain species of fish carry hollow organs on the head which house colonies of bacteria. The bacteria thrive off secretions from special glands. In return for this hospitality they glow in the dark and the luminous patches which they create attract prey and serve as recognition and warning signals between the fish in the perpetual darkness of the ocean deeps. The divisions between parasitism, commensalism and symbiosis are often blurred, and indeed the role of an organism may change with respect to its host. But the more it helps its host the more likely it is to be tolerated undisturbed.

The bounty which we offer unknowingly on the surface of our skins does not go unrewarded. Recently it has been shown that not all the bacteria on our skin are simply commensal. For example, work at the Westminster Hospital Medical School has shown that there are varieties which thrive in the conditions of a wound, but they produce an antibiotic which defends us against infection by harmful strains of bacteria. The disadvantage of this helpful conduct is that the wound then heals and removes their favoured habitat, so they are found only on one in five of us. A really successful symbiont is indispensable. If we were entirely to give up breast-feeding babies the future of the cow would be assured for as long as the human race survived.

To the microbe the 2 square metres of skin of the prettiest girl is no more than a habitat with a surprisingly diverse set of microclimates, from the moist tropical forests of the armpits to the cool arid deserts of the back of the forearm. The complex flora and fauna which inhabit these different areas behave according to strict ecological considerations – just as they do in a forest or a plain. In this complicated world in miniature, they depend both on each other and on us, and however hard we may try to get rid of them a few individuals will always survive to breed a new colony. Even more important is the fact that the existing population will deter the arrival of dangerous new-comers.

The importance of this stable relationship can be seen from the results of a rather macabre experiment. If a culture of typhoid germs, the bacterium *Salmonella typhi*, is smeared on the skin and then regularly sampled every few minutes, within twenty minutes there are very few bacteria still alive. A culture simultaneously spread on a glass microscope slide will live and remain active, and a third smear on a human corpse behaves much more like the smear on glass.

Basically the skin is an inhospitable place for bacteria which are not specifically evolved to live there; it is salty and acid, and the surface constantly breaks away to float off into the air. It is, in fact, a most effective barrier between our inner tissues and the world, but it is quite wrong to think of the skin as uninhabited. Its population has developed to take advantage of the conditions present, and secure in its ecological integrity the established organisms strive jealously to maintain the *status quo*. We may have from as few as fifteen to as many as three million bacteria on each square centimetre of our skins. While our skin is intact they are neither harmful nor avoidable, and no amount of scrub-bing will get them off a surgeon's hands. Yet the skin is probably the least studied of all the organs of our bodies. There are two fairly obvious reasons for this: doctors have always been more interested in states of disease than health, and given adequate nutrition and reasonable care the skin has quite remarkable self-healing properties; and secondly, the inhabitants of our skinny world are so tiny that most of them can only be seen under the high powers of a microscope. Indeed there is still no really satisfactory visual way of recognizing one type from another.

The whole concept of 'the ecology of the human skin' is probably due to the work of one woman, Professor Mary Marples, who began her scientific life as an ecologist long before the word was familiar to fellow scientists, let alone in Fleet Street. Moving to New Zealand with her husband she trained as a bacteriologist and in 1965 published a vast tome with the above title. I must at once acknowledge my debt to her for the information and the encouragement she gave me to make the BBC television programme which gave rise to this book. She gave me two telling examples of why the population of our skin is so often ignored.

The rod-shaped bacteria which inhabit our skin are two to four microns in length, while the cocci or spherical forms are about one micron in diameter. A micron is a thousandth of a millimetre. A millimetre is clearly visible on a ruler, so if the coccus was enlarged a thousand times it could be readily seen and would look like the head of a pin. But if its human host were enlarged to match he would be more than a mile in height. Another way of picturing the relative sizes of man and a member of his normal flora is to imagine the man enlarged until his feet were at Land's End and the top of his head at John o'Groats. A coccus enlarged to the same scale would be about the size of a half-grown lamb in one of the fields which he would cover.

To the same scale a fragment of skin would be about the size of a farmyard, and our slightest movement whirls countless numbers of these into the air. Experiments in sterile chambers have shown that an individual sheds a million of these skin rafts into the air in forty minutes, each carrying on them their passive passengers. Undoubtedly they are an important source of infection in operating theatres, as the skin scales are tiny enough to pass easily through clothing. Imagine then the cataclysm on this miniature landscape wrought by the simple action of undressing, with millions of bacteria condemned to an arid death. After all, that grey dust on top of the wardrobe or in the bag of your vacuum-cleaner is almost all shed skin.

Before going on to see how the skin works as a self-maintaining system it is interesting to compare it with other living systems. Ordinary soil gains its organic material from dead plants, the skin from secretions and the slow migration of new scales from below. Both the soil and the skin surface are dead and in both cases the highest populations of living organisms are below the surface in the root layer and the hair follicle. Estimates of the number of bacteria and fungi in the soil vary from a million to a thousand million in each gram, and since over half a million bacteria have been estimated to be present in a milligram of scurf (a clump of skin scales) the population comes well within the range for fertile soil. Since we do not normally start to grow mushrooms under our armpits, we can see at once that our skin provides conditions which are inhospitable to all but an extremely small number of species, which are present in astronomical numbers.

The study of ecology is the interrelation of the interactions of all living and non-living things, and in proper terms it must relate to the study of all life on the planet, but by drawing a boundary line around an entity such as a field, or a wood, or a pond, the ecologist can consider the processes and substances which cross the boundary as well as what goes on inside it, and make a meaningful analysis of the *status quo*. The most important characteristic of any such system which has natural boundaries is that it is self-sustaining. The competitive forces of population growth and food supply finally come into balance. Under stable climatic conditions a wood will support a given number of pairs of owls, dependent on the number of mice and shrews, in turn dependent on the supply of seeds and insects and controlled by the number of weasels. The animal population will also be related to the number of trees and plants, and the fertility of the soil. Each species forms a link in an intricate interconnected pattern of relationships with other species and with the inanimate surroundings. This is precisely what happens on the landscape of our skins, which like the pond or wood is an eco-system. Just as it came as a shock to farmers to find that the use of Dieldrin as a pesticidal seed-dressing resulted in the near extinction of the peregrine falcon from the British Isles, so doctors at first found it hard to believe that prescribing tablets of the antibiotic tetracycline caused marked and not always beneficial changes in the microbial population of our skins. We upset the natural balance at our peril, however unsavoury the thought of a teeming skin may be.

Our skin makes up about 16 per cent of our total body weight and varies in thickness from 1 millimetre on the eyelids to 3 millimetres between the shoulder blades and on the palms and soles, although people who habitually go barefoot may have soles 1 centimetre thick. It is formed of two layers; beneath the visible epidermis lies the dermis which is the major producer of raw material for the eco-system. The latter contains the nerves and blood and lymph vessels and into it penetrate the sweat glands, sebaceous glands and hair follicles. None of the normally resident organisms reaches the dermis unless the skin is damaged or diseased, so the epidermis is our main interest.

The surface of our skin is dead, and seen at a high magnification it looks like nothing so much as an irregular patch of curling cornflakes of an astonishingly rough and disagreeable appearance. These tough horny flakes, properly called squames, are the desiccated remnants of skin cells which are constantly being formed at the base of the epidermis and travel slowly outwards. It seems that most of the cell division which forms the skin cells takes place at night and it takes forty to fifty-six days for a newly formed cell to reach the surface. By that time it has died, not from contact with the air, but from the formation of keratin fibres, the same horny material which makes up our hair and finger-nails. For the last two weeks the cells lie in what is called the *stratum corneum* where they are dead, flat, and firmly attached to each other to form the barrier we know as our skin. One of its most important properties is that it restricts the movement of moisture in either direction. If this layer is damaged or rubbed away it stimulates the basal cells to reproduce more quickly. Quite how this happens nobody knows, and it is one of the most intriguing research topics in medical science. Uncontrolled growth is a feature of cancer cells, and until it is discovered how normal cells know when to switch their reproduction on or off, there is little hope of learning why cancer cells escape this control. One possible clue is that cortisone slows up the division of skin cells.

The shedding apparatus is one of our effective weapons against infection: the more our skin gets damaged or dirty the more it flakes away. Even the most stubborn stains on a finger 'wear off' after a time as the affected cells are replaced from below. But this turnover of the surface does not remove the normal population of micro-organisms as they are in the crevices leading down deeper into the *stratum corneum* where there is a better supply of food substances, and also in the various glands and holes which penetrate the surface.

From the sweat glands oozes a salty liquid 99·5 per cent water. Half the rest is salt, but it also carries nutrient chemicals. The ebb and flow of these salty pits is clearly a considerable influence on the life nearby and depends on two kinds of stimuli. The sweat glands on the palms and soles react only to mental processes like fright or pain or mental arithmetic under stress. Sweat appears within two minutes of the presence of adrenalin in the blood, and the sweaty palm was almost certainly evolved as an aid to grip in fight or flight situations. The labourer still spits on his hands before gripping a shovel. The other normal stimulus for sweating is heat. Any temperature above 32°C will cause sweating.

The sweat ducts grow inwards from the epidermis in the embryo and when they reach the base of the dermis they form a jumbled coil of tube lined with secreting cells. Each gland can double its water production in response to a rise in temperature of 7°–8°C, and evaporation then contributes a substantial cooling effect. A sweat gland can produce about 150 millilitres of water a day. Four-fifths of our water loss can be through the sweat glands and the damper the skin becomes, the more permeable it is and the more water passes through it. An adult has from seventy sweat glands per square centimetre on his back to over four hundred per square centimetre on his palms and soles. Since all glands are present at birth, and the surface area of a child is much smaller, the glands are much more tightly packed and sweating that much more profuse – as any mother who has picked up her over-heated baby can tell. Tiny babies, on the other hand, cannot sweat at all. General sweating can also be caused by eating spicy food, perhaps the reason why the further one travels towards the equator in India, the hotter the curries become.

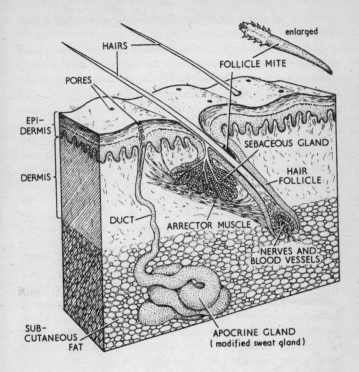

HAIRS

enlarged

FOLLICLE MITE

PORES

EPI-
DERMIS

DERMIS

SEBACEOUS GLAND

HAIR
FOLLICLE

DUCT

ARRECTOR MUSCLE

NERVES AND
BLOOD VESSELS

SUB-
CUTANEOUS
FAT

APOCRINE GLAND
( modified sweat gland )

*Diagram of skin section*

Survivors of the Raj will be interested to know that a study on Japanese born and living in the tropics showed that they had nearly three million sweat glands each while those living in a temperate climate had few more than two million. This does not imply that they had aquired more sweat glands through being hot, because this is impossible genetically, but instead dormant sweat glands had been turned on in childhood. A British Army study in Aden also showed that soldiers became acclimatized to heat by greatly increasing the amount of water they drank after a fortnight in the desert; this increased their sweat production. Considering that we have so many, it is astonishing that the eccrine sweat gland was only discovered by science about fifty years ago.

The other form of sweat gland which causes a special local environment is the apocrine gland. These are ten times as wide as sweat gland openings and exude a milky secretion into hair follicles. They are found in the armpits, groin, around the nipples and umbilicus, and a few on the face. They are said to be more common on women than men, and although their secretion has no marked smell initially, it is broken down by bacteria to form the socially abhorrent BO. In fact there is a good deal of evidence to suggest that far from being socially repellent, apocrine secretions may well contain pheromones, the attractant hormones which invite the interest of the opposite sex.

Apocrine glands react to sex hormones, and armpit sweating starts during adolescence. Male hormones encourage apocrine secretion and female hormones inhibit it (both men and women produce both kinds of hormones). The same happens in many animals, such as the rabbit. The buck rabbit has three kinds of apocrine glands, on the chin, in the anal area, and in the groin. He marks a female by 'chinning' in the same way that he marks his territory by rubbing sticks or ground and will chase away a female marked by another male. Marked droppings are similar territorial boundary posts and the anal and chin glands are thought to produce the same substance.

If the secretion from the groin glands is presented to a doe, she immediately adopts behaviour characteristic of mating. In other words it is a pheromone.

Man's apocrine glands may well have had the same function during evolution, and it's well worth while noting the markedly different attitudes of the Anglo-Saxons and the French to female underarm hair. The beauty editor of a famous fashion magazine once showed me a sample perfume sent her by a major manufacturer which, they specifically explained, was compounded to mimic the smell of the sweat of a young girl. It never became a commercial product, but it does seem more logical to entice the human male with a female odour than to exploit the anal glands of a civet cat as many perfumes do.

The most obvious feature interrupting the surface of the skin is the hair follicle, a deep pocket of epidermis acting as a sheath to the root of the hair. Hairs always grow at an angle to the surface so that there is a smooth flow of hair across every part of the skin. Each follicle has its own arrector muscle which can pull the hair into a more upright position, easily recognizable as 'gooseflesh'. Many people are sceptical of stories of scalp hair standing on end, other than by the effects of static electricity, but I can vouch for the following hair-raising anecdote.

A cameraman friend of mine had been filming a fully grown tiger at the BBC studios at Ealing for a children's programme. The lights were hot and during the tea-break both tiger and cameraman had a snooze. The tiger was clipped by a chain lead to a metal post and the cameraman sat on a pile of chairs beside it, careful to keep just beyond range of its claws. On to this unusual but tranquil scene came an electrician who had not been working on the set, and seeing the cameraman and tiger together, with a shout of 'Yah Jim, you can't fool me, it's stuffed!' strode up to the tiger and jabbed it hard in the ribs with two fingers. With a roar the tiger leaped into the air and the chain fell from its neck. It then tore in a streak of yellow and orange round the studio before bursting through the doors into the passage where it had a noisy encounter with the laden tea-trolley. Meanwhile the short black curly hair on the electrician's scalp stood on end, appearing to uncurl itself like a paper party-whistle. The same cool cameraman later cornered the tiger and it was returned to its cage without injury to life or limb.

Why does man, of all the land mammals, appear to be naked? The answer, claimed Charles Darwin, is that men for countless millennia have preferred women who exposed their charms to view. By mating selectively with the ones with less visible body hair the children became slowly more naked. (A rather similar process is happening now on some of the West Indian islands where a fair skin and straight hair are prestigious and are given a genetic advantage by colour biased marriages.) A less romantic explanation is that loss of hair and multiplication of sweat glands are an adaptation to the hot plains of the tropics made when man left the shade of the jungle. Only a thatch on top was necessary to prevent his head from addling in the midday sun.

Surprisingly, a woman has as many active hair follicles as a man, even on her cheeks. The difference is that the fine hair on a girl's face is vellus hair. In fact we have as many hairs growing on our foreheads and cheeks as a monkey has in the same area of pelt on his back. The difference is the quality rather than quantity. Each hair follicle is able to make three or more different kinds of hair. The first to appear is lanugo, the long colourless silky-soft hair sometimes seen on premature babies. This is usually superseded by vellus hair a month or two before birth, but a late change-over can result in a blotchy infant. Vellus hair remains throughout adulthood on our upper cheeks, ears, most of our bodies, and limbs. It is often colourless and rarely grows longer than an inch. The hairs of the scalp, eyebrows and eyelashes, in contrast, are much coarser and more pigmented, and in the case of the scalp, longer. This coarser hair and the hair which comes with puberty in the armpits, groin, and on the chest is called terminal hair. Hair follicles do not increase in number with age, so the density of hair on a child is again higher than that on an adult, but each follicle goes through a cycle of activity. The cycle of hair growth followed by withering and a rest period when no hair is produced is necessary to restrict the length of the shorter hairs, and to replace damaged hair. The life of a vellus hair is about four and a half months, while scalp hair lives for three to five years. It is ironic that hair plucked out regrows most rapidly on the eyebrows, one of the few areas where it is removed by women, and on the chin, the area where it is mowed down daily by men. In each case the rate of growth is about a third of a millimetre a day. If you avoided your barber for a year, your hair would grow by about 12 centimetres, and it takes six years before it is long enough to sit on. Sikhs and followers of Samson who never cut their hair will never find themselves tripping over it, as the average maximum length of locks is about 1 metre. Some unfortunates, however, can never grow their hair long as it only attains a short length before it succumbs to the daily shedding of thirty to sixty hairs.

An average scalp contains from 100 to 150 thousand hairs, so this loss from the temporary inactivity of follicles is negligible, but many a dupe has been scalped in a baldness clinic as a result of far less evidence on his comb.

We all have bald palms and soles and finger and toe ends, but the sad truth is that 58 per cent of men are substantially bald at the age of fifty. One in five is very bald by thirty. There are two main types of male baldness or *alopecia*; in one the hair loss begins before the age of thirty and is extensive by forty, in the other it starts later. Both are caused by a dominant gene. It is not a sex-linked gene as in the blood disease haemophilia, it just affects men more severely. I have an ancestor called Oswald the Bald, who was one of the Welsh kings. Although sixty generations have been laid to rest the relentless inheritance, even though it passes through the female as well as male line, still harvests my own brow.

Aristotle pointed out that boys never go bald, nor women, nor do castrated men, an observation verified by a French dermatologist in the harem of the Sultan of Turkey! The inference is that baldness depends on the presence of the male testicular hormone, testosterone. There is thus only one cure for baldness which most men would think twice before undertaking – castration. This was confirmed by James Hamilton in 1941 in a study of the male inmates of a mental asylum in Kansas where all too recently the barbaric practice of sterilization was carried out in the guise of therapy. Patients who had been castrated before puberty were injected with testosterone. It was found that those who had baldness in the family promptly began to lose their hair. When the testosterone was stopped the recession stopped. To be made experimentally bald when you have no chance of saying 'No' would appear to add insult to injury.

Some forms of patchy baldness, accounting for less than 5 per cent of cases, may occur after ill health or operations, and may clear up spontaneously or with treatment.

For the benefit of any sceptic reading this chapter I repeat that at the time of writing there is *no* cure for male-pattern baldness which leaves the testes intact. Ever since Paracelsus, the founder of pharmacy, pates have been anointed with chemicals which had, if anything, even less effect than the viper-oil, bats' ears and myrrh of the Egyptians. But clearly there is a huge fortune awaiting the lucky man to discover why the follicles seize up, and many big pharmaceutical firms have research projects under way. Perhaps a clue for them might be the report that a gas-fitter in Stevenage who had been bald for sixteen years found his hair returning after stopping leaks in North Sea natural gas pipes. Meanwhile, hope dies hard; when workers in a chicken dung manure factory reported hair returning to their balding heads, 10 000 optimists wrote in with orders for the product.

More seriously speaking, two Russian scientists in 1974 said they had found a silicon organic compound which caused the hair on guinea-pigs to grow six times as long as normal. Since then they have been experimenting with both mink and bald pates. Success with either would seem good business.

Whilst men become obsessed by a lack of hair, women go to the opposite extreme. Not so long ago trichologists used X-rays to remove surplus hair. It worked splendidly, but the heavy doses of radiation also caused cancer. It was only in 1949 that the last such machine was switched off in America. Women, however, can take comfort from the fact that the rate of hair growth slows by a quarter from the thirteenth week of pregnancy. But sometimes childbirth introduces a disconcerting temporary moult. Abnormal shedding sometimes follows operations or great stress. Ten weeks after one American was condemned to death, he started to lose more than 1 000 hairs a day and was soon completely bald. His sentence was commuted, and he regrew his hair.

The amount of facial hair of different races varies considerably. Some Indians of the Andes have no beards at all, and while the Caucasian male reaches his beard-producing peak between the ages of thirty and forty, and sprouts 40 milligrams of beard per chin-day, his Japanese competitor has on average only half the area of beard, does not reach full production until sixty, and then only reaps 12 milligrams. This must be the reason why we have not yet been flooded with Japanese-made razor-blades. Those who indulge in multiracial saunas may also have noticed that white girls grow four times as much underarm hair as yellow ones.

Negro hair tends to be flat in cross-section, where curly or straight hair is oval to round. These flat or ribbon-shaped hairs do not lie flat on a level surface but tend to spiral. This leads to knots which can be a painful hazard of long Afro hair styles.

Hair grows from a lump called the papilla at the base of the follicle, and by the time the hair has grown to the skin surface, the cells which compose the bulk of the hair, the cortex, have become full of keratin and are long and spindle-shaped. In a mature hair the cortex looks like a bundle of fibres tightly cemented together surrounded by a sheath of overlapping cuticle cells like curved tiles. One of the hazards of back-combing hair is that it prises up the edge of these cuticle cells and the hair then splits or becomes invaded with yeast cells. Hair-spray simply glues individual hairs together where they cross, and in spite of claims that it brushes out, spray inevitably leaves a residue on the uneven surface of hair. Once hair has been damaged it can never repair itself since, of course, it is dead; but hair is very resistant to damage by micro-organisms. Animal remains and mummies demonstrate that it can survive for thousands of years without decay, and clearly if scalp hair remains on the head for three to five years a degree of resistance to decay is essential. Usually it is destroyed in the end by the attack of fungi.

About two-thirds of the way up the hair follicle is found the opening of the sebaceous gland. This exudes the oily liquid called sebum which mixes easily with sweat and forms a film over the surface of the skin near each hair follicle. Its main function appears to be a conditioner for keratin, it delays moisture loss and keeps out foreign matter, but the presence of the oily, salty, slightly acid surface film is of great importance to the life of our bacteria and fungi. Sebum is formed by the disintegration of fat-laden cells inside the bag-like sebaceous gland. We have no such glands on the palms and soles and their size bears no relationship to the coarseness of the hair in the follicle. Indeed the greatest production of sebum occurs on the forehead and scalp. In general more sebum is produced on the mid-line of the chest and back than towards the sides. If the sebum film is removed by a solvent it is replaced within two to four hours and there is a good deal of debate among physiologists as to how the gland knows when to secrete more, as it shows no tendency to flood the surface once the film is formed. Girls only produce about half as much sebum as men, and the production is linked to their monthly hormonal cycle. The hormone, oestrogen, reduces sebum output so girls on the Pill produce less sebum as well as apocrine secretion, and it is interesting to speculate whether this is one of the causes of reported loss of libido on the part of their husbands. Babies have active sebaceous glands because of the presence of androgens (male hormones) from the mother but the activity subsides again in childhood until reaching full production at puberty.

The skin must contain 10 per cent water to remain flexible and too dry an atmosphere or too much soap causes flaking and cracking – chapping. Moisturizing creams, which fill so many advertising pages in women's magazines, are either emollients which delay water loss, usually with a greasy film, or are humectants which draw water from the air but also from the skin. According to the Consumers' Association magazine *Which?* the most expensive brand is 150 times the cost of the cheapest, but they found that people could not tell the difference between cheap and expensive brands unless told.

One of the more unusual habitats of the skin is the outer ear, where the apocrine glands have been modified to produce ear-wax (cerumen). The internal ear, especially in children, is one of the most frequent places where infection takes place from bacteria which are normally harmless colonizers of the nose.

By way of a summary it is helpful to reconsider the eco-system from the viewpoint of a bacterium ensconced on your forearm. Again the illustration comes from Mary Marples.

In 1 square centimetre there will be about 100 hair follicles and 220 sweat glands. If this area is multiplied by 10 000 it would be 100 metres square with occasional hairs about every

30 metres; each one springing from a greasy pit and having about the diameter of a moderate-sized tree trunk. Scattered over this surface are the irregular openings of the sweat glands with salt-encrusted rims, about the diameter of a drain-pipe liable to disgorge droplets of water several metres across at the slightest rise in temperature. In this open savanna-like landscape the huge majority of the inhabitants are bacteria which on the same scale would be 5 centimetres long, the size of a small shrew. There would be about 150 000 shrews in our 100-metre square, about 15 per square metre, and they would have the disconcerting habit of stretching and then breaking into two individuals before your eyes.

# 4

# Bacteria, Viruses and Yeasts

*Adam had 'em.*
    'ON THE ANTIQUITY OF PARASITES'
By repute the oldest poem in the English language

It is all a question of scale. Fleas have parasites too, and bacteria can parasitize the parasites of fleas, and viruses can parasitize the same bacteria. As Jonathan Swift put it:

> So naturalists observe, a flea
> Hath smaller fleas that on him prey;
> And these have smaller fleas to bite 'em,
> And so proceed *ad infinitum*.

Our parasites also scarcely qualify for inclusion as we have so few of them. A man would be thought pretty unfortunate to have to tolerate twenty fleas in his bed, but as many as 3340 have been recovered from one grey squirrel's nest. Life under such conditions would seem to be quite intolerable yet the host can become dependent on his parasites. One hedgehog which had 980 fleas removed from it later died, possibly because its bloodstream had become so accustomed to the parasitic bloodletting that it killed itself with antitoxins. It is helpful to remember that in Nature friend and foe, cause and effect, are not always easily distinguishable. This is equally true of the microorganisms which inhabit our skins.

To analyse any ecological system it helps to divide the living participants into groups according to what they do. First there are the producers, which in the countryside are generally green plants that turn inorganic material into organic by using the energy of the sun. Then there are the consumer animals which get their energy instead by feeding on plants or each other. And lastly there are the decomposing fungi and bacteria – 'germs' which break down dead plants and animals and return their component substances to the soil.

From childhood we are brought up to believe that germs are evil. Prejudice, carefully fostered by disinfectant advertisers, paints them as demons to be pursued from the four corners of our lives with liberal applications of expensive sanitary products. There cannot be a surer way of making money than to convince the public that they must buy your potion to pour it down the drain! While some germs are indeed dangerous, there are many which we need in order to stay alive. Fortunately for us the overall effect of our disinfectants on the total population of germs is negligible.

It is illuminating instead to consider what would happen without the presence of the humble invisible bacterium. The continuity of the carbon and nitrogen cycles between plants and animals would cease. Starved of their essential constituents all living things would eventually die out and the world would become a perpetual museum of everlasting corpses.

We associate putrefaction with death, yet it is caused by an enormous abundance of life, of millions of bacteria. Far from being a menace they restore to the earth the raw materials necessary for more life. In one sense bacteria are the fount of all life, yet because the bacterium has no skeleton or bony shell its history is eliminated from the fossil record and essential though it is, its exact place beside our unicellular ancestors in the primeval seas cannot be confirmed or refuted.

On the surface of our skins, our bodies are the producers and only the follicle mite (see Chapter 5) is a consumer. The ecological circle of production, consumption and decay is only completed once our skin has been shed, or when we die. Our other animal fauna are parasites and in medical literature are not included as normal inhabitants, even though they may be present in a majority of a given group of individuals as is all too often the case. The fact that they can modify the local environment is obvious from the readiness with which bacteria invade the wounds made by scabies and lice to cause impetigo. By causing our death, the typhus-carrying louse, or the plague flea which has fed on a dying rat, destroy the hope of survival of millions of micro-organisms dependent on us.

Apart from the danger of being wafted off into the air, or being washed or scratched away, the organisms on our skin live a comfortable life. Most other bacteria however have to spend their lives alternately heated by the sun and chilled at night. At the top of equatorial mountains the temperature can range from − 30°C at night to 30 or 40°C in the sun at noon. On our skins there are no seasons and no daily variation, so the temperature range is comparatively small.

Our body heat comes both from muscular exertion and the continuous chemical reactions taking place at the cellular level throughout our tissues, but it is not evenly distributed. Habitual sharers of double-beds will know that a cold spouse is always accompanied by even colder feet and hands. The reason is that the extremities of the body are used as temperature-regulating radiators. If the body is hot the blood circulation in the extremities is opened up and heat is literally pumped away to the fingers and toes by the heart. Since they have a large surface area they are much better able to disperse heat than the body, especially as they are not covered with hair or clothes. Conversely if the brain senses cold, it sends messages for the capillaries in the hands and feet to be shut down, sometimes resulting in white fingers or even frostbite, and heat loss from the vital organs is delayed at the price of cold feet. Despairing wives could make use of the fact that a hearty meal has been shown to cause a significant and prolonged rise in the skin temperature of toes even of those sleeping in arctic conditions.

Body temperature will rarely drop below 25°C, without triggering a fit of shivering, and since the upper limit is about 35°C, bacteria on the trunk have to endure a temperature change of only 10°.

## Viruses

The smallest live inhabitants of our skins, the viruses, are also inevitably the least studied and there are really few useful observations that can be made in a non-specialist book. They are the smallest form of life and can only reproduce by entering a living cell of an animal or plant where they trick the cell into making more of their own genetic material. The viruses multiply in this way inside the cell until it bursts, releasing them to colonize other cells. They are visible only with an electron microscope, as their size, about a tenth that of a small bacterium, is too small compared with the wavelength of light to be seen with any lens. The virus which first concerns us is the *Herpes virus hominis* which causes 'cold sores' in response to any lowering of the resistance of the host by infection, sunburn or stress. It is now thought that the virus retreats from the skin surface up the nerve axons to colonize the nerve centres. The skin infection subsides and all seems well until some lowering of the individual's immunity allows them to come teeming down the axon to cause trouble again. More than 90 per cent of the population carry *Herpes virus* and it is usually caught in childhood. Once infected, it is carried for life, and the general effect of its presence is unknown. It is disconcerting to find that cancer research raises the suspicion that it might be involved in the outbreak of some cancers.

Warts are benign, but often provoking and difficult to remove. These are caused, not by washing in water in which eggs have been boiled, but by the papova virus, which stimulates irregular growth of the epidermis. Because of the shape of a wart and the fact that it is relatively cut off from the bloodstream it is not easily attacked by the body's defensive army of cells and it may have an unpredictable future.

Just because the lifetime of warts is so unpredictable folk remedies for them abound; moles' blood, fasting saliva, water collected from hollows in the bark of poplar trees, cobwebs, the white cushiony lining of broad-bean pods, boiled roots of teasel, or the caustic juices of the greater celandine, or the St John's wort; all are supposed to be cures. Casting spells or hexing are equally recommended for the credulous. If you ask the moon she will waft them away, or a friend can buy them with a penny (a new penny?). It is claimed to be especially efficacious to rub them with steak, all the better if it is stolen first and buried in secret afterwards, and for the brave, I am told, one infallible method is to stick a pin into the centre of the wart and then heat the head of the pin until it is red hot with a candle (but sterilize the pin first). The cowardly, on the other hand, have been advised to rub the wart with a slug and then to impale the wretched mollusc on a thorn.

Modern cures are almost as bizarre. Warts are frozen off with liquid nitrogen or carbon dioxide, vibrated off with ultrasound, irradiated with X-rays, parched with electro-desiccation, fooled with placebo therapy and even removed with hypnosis. People have been inoculated with vaccinea virus in the hope of a cure – with a danger of a serious systemic reaction, and the vitamin pedlars have plugged vitamin A cream. Mostly, the truth is that warts go if left well alone, and their disappearance is only connected with any of the folk remedies by coincidence. The successes are reported, but not the failures.

Scientific survey supports the belief that they go of their own accord. One British study followed the progress of 2000 patients with warts on the soles of their feet. Ninety-seven per cent of untreated cases recovered spontaneously while only 84 per cent of patients who had been treated lost their warts. In other words the best way to get rid of warts is to leave them well alone. Two-thirds of all warts disappear within a year or two and almost all vanish within three years.

Warts are quite definitely contagious; the virus tends to invade slightly damaged skin, and then will spread to various members of a family. They can be caught on the feet, where they are especially awkward and painful, from contaminated floors. But the family pets are safe: human wart virus will not infect hamsters or horses.

It is possible that the connection with egg-water is not entirely erroneous. One American dermatologist noticed a high incidence of warts on the hands of meat cutters working at a meat packing plant. In reply to a questionnaire he found that 44 per cent of meat cutters had warts while only 24 per cent of automobile workers had them. Possibly meat or poultry have the capacity to transmit the virus to man. Equally possible meat packers damage the skin on their hands more often and so are more liable to infection.

Another intriguing aspect of viruses is that when we have had a virus disease in our system the virus may get into the living skin cells in the dermis and then remain in the desiccated cell squames which are shed. Normally virus infections are considered contagious through droplets carried in the air (foot-and-mouth disease usually spreads downwind of the initial outbreak) and we all know that coughs and sneezes spread diseases. It may well be that scratching your head can be just as anti-social.

## Bacteria

The bacteria which so dominate life on the skin are the simplest form of free-living life, consisting of one cell. (Viruses are incapable of reproducing outside a host cell.) Although they do not contain chlorophyll they are usually classified with plants rather than with animals, but they do not fit easily into either description. They are small spheres or rounded rods and only a few kinds are able to move themselves by rippling a fringe of mobile hairs. Mostly they are passive creatures simply jostling each other out of the way as they multiply by dividing in two. They gather their food and energy requirements from their surroundings, but it is believed that those which are responsible for diseases such as tuberculosis, diphtheria, typhoid and pneumonia are strains which have lost the ability to synthesize some essential nutrients which must be supplied by the unfortunate host. One result of this is the more specialized a bacterium becomes for a parasitic existence, the more infectious is the disease which it causes.

Bacteria are alive and exploiting dead organic matter almost everywhere. The numbers are so huge as to be beyond our comprehension. Our intimacy with them may be uncomfortable to those obsessed with cleanliness, but even the most radiantly antiseptic housewife will be covered in thousands of millions of them. They thrive, as the saying goes, in every nook of Granny. And not just on the outside; half of the bulk of our faeces are the dead bodies of bacteria which live in the gut.

A bacterium can divide every twenty minutes, so under ideal conditions a single organism can multiply to 512 in three hours, or a million in under eight hours. It is this astonishing ability to reproduce which has made the bacterium such a successful form of life. Varieties have adapted to every condition on earth where there is moisture, they can live in the hot springs surrounding geysers and thrive in the refrigerator. They can also survive being freeze-dried, indeed this is a method used to transfer cultures by ordinary post from lab to lab. Because of this ability they have been carried up into space and survived that.

Because of the way they rule our lives, bacteria have been extensively studied. But once again those on the skin have had little attention paid to them except in the last ten years. They do not normally cause disease, and since bacteriologists, like all of us, prefer to do work which is considered important they have concentrated on the dramatic disease-causing organisms. Only recently has this tendency been reversed in a few teaching hospitals and medical schools where it has come to be realized that the behaviour of our normal bacterial population may be just as important to health as the onslaught of diseases.

The smallest mote of dust that you can see in a sunbeam is about 12 microns across, and the diameter of one of the spherical bacteria about 1 micron (a thousandth of a millimetre). A large one will be about 5 microns long. Moreover the average life of one bacterium is only twenty minutes, so bacteria have been traditionally studied not in isolation but in colonies.

From the very first work of Pasteur and Koch, bacteria have been studied by their effects on ourselves and our surroundings rather than for what they are in themselves or how they live, and except in specialist laboratories working on their structure this attitude continues. At first they were classified by their actions in producing fermentation or disease, then by their shape. A spherical bacterium was called a coccus (a berry) and a cigar-shaped one a bacillus (a stick). Unfortunately strains of bacteria which appear identical can be either harmless or lethal. Once when Pasteur was politely told that a bacterium he had called a coccus was in reality a bacillus, he retorted sharply: 'If you only knew how little difference that makes to me!'

In the middle of the last century Pasteur had shown that bacteria were far more numerous in cities than in the country-side and rare in rooms where the dust was undisturbed. They are a ubiquitous accompaniment to our lives, at one extreme exist-ing in hailstones, and at another they often enter our blood. One famous experiment in the 1920s showed that the air of the fashionable Paris *salon* supported five million bacteria to the cubic metre. Since we breathe about a third of a cubic foot of air the gallery-goers were inhaling 60 000 bacteria with every breath.

Pasteur's pioneering studies of bacteria had begun on fermen-tation of wine and beer and he continued to grow his bacteria in liquids. It was Koch who made the great advance of using solid media, at first potatoes or gelatin and later agar extracted from seaweed, which allowed colonies to grow which could be identified as specific by their appearance. Koch then discovered that certain chemicals would stain some bacteria and not others, and a system of classification began.

The basic division between types of bacteria are according to their response to the Gram stain named after the Danish bacteriologist Hans Gram. Some bacteria stain dark purple and are referred to as gram positive, and others which stain red are called gram negative. The distinction is of use not because it demonstrates different chemical characteristics of the two types, but because it happens to distinguish their structure and disease-causing capabilities as well.

The skin is colonized chiefly by gram positive bacteria and the intestines by the gram negative variety. The gram positive skin bacteria can be subdivided into different groups. First there are the small spherical cocci which are dependent on oxygen. They are classed within the family known as Micrococcaceae and chiefly belong to the genera *Staphylococcus, Micrococcus* and *Sarcina*. But the whole categorization process appears to a layman like myself to be in a state of chaos with one research worker unable to repeat the results of another. On one point there is, however, general agreement: that the types of *Staphylococcus* that are dangerous to man if they invade his tissues can be identified because they have the capacity to coagulate human plasma in the test-tube. The worst of these grows colonies of a golden colour and is called *Staphylococcus aureus*. Usually its destructive propensities are confined to generating pimples and boils, and in a large number of individuals it is a permanent resident of the nose and perineum (the area between the genitals and the anus). It has however been described as 'the most uniformly fatal of all blood infections'. Nevertheless the majority of cocci are at worst harmless and at best beneficial to us, and they play an active role against invasion by their sinister cousins.

The second group of gram positive bacteria are rod-shaped and can be divided into three groups, all called diphtheroids. The first species thrives without oxygen in the depths of the hair follicle and because of its association with acne is called *Corynebacterium acnes*. The other diphtheroids need oxygen and can be divided because some will grow well without fatty nutrients, such as sebum, whilst the others need them.

So much misery has been caused by acne, and such fortunes have been made selling 'cures' that I shall discuss it in more detail in a later chapter, but in general the diphtheroids are considered to be harmless. This is probably for lack of any evidence to quote against them rather than because they have been exonerated, because very little research has so far been carried out. If it was discovered that they had a crucial role to play in some military activity no doubt money would flood in to sponsor research projects. As it is they remain unknown.

Within the large families of cocci and diphtheroids there are countless numbers of different species. The sub-groups of *Staphylococcus* can only be told apart by the viruses that parasitize them called phage viruses. One strain of bacteria can be told from another according to whether it is killed or not by specific viruses, and it is on the basis of this differentiation that a proper system of designation and description of these bacteria is slowly being built up.

A few gram negative strains of bacteria also appear on the skin especially on the feet of children and men. Some of them are capable of movement, swimming along with their hair-like *flagellae*. If the normal flora of the skin is maltreated the gram negative bacteria from the gut can re-colonize the skin instead and I will have more to say about this later.

A baby in the womb is sterile, but in the process of being born it picks up its first bacteria from its mother. If, on the other hand, it is born by a Caesarean operation, it will remain sterile, and animals such as pigs have been reared in totally sterile conditions to study the effect of different bacteria on their health and rate of growth.

Just because the skin of a baby is not yet colonized it will be extremely receptive to infection, and its skin will slowly be populated more or less on a first-come-first-served basis. A typical experiment on bacterial numbers in the armpit showed 6000 bacteria per square centimetre one day after birth, rising to 24 000 by the fifth day and then stabilizing around 81 000 after the ninth day of the baby's life. Once the resident population has built up it makes it far harder for the pathogens (the disease-causing organisms) to survive. For example, it has been shown that if one phage-type *Staphylococcus* is found in the nose of a baby, it is rare to find another. One study showed that a nurse in a maternity ward carried one phage-type of the dangerous *Staphylococcus aureus* in her nose. She handled thirty-seven babies within twenty-four hours of their being born; nearly a quarter of them caught her bacteria. But of the thirty-one babies more than twenty-four hours old which she handled repeatedly, not one was colonized. Instead 81 per cent of the second group were colonized with a different *Staphylococcus aureus*.

In San Francisco attempts have been made to stop babies being colonized by dangerous *Staphylococcus* by getting in first with an inoculation of a phage-type known to be harmless. But following the initial experiments it was decided that too little was known about the behaviour of *Staphylococcus* to risk repeating the work.

The type and number of bacteria are closely controlled by the exact habitat on the skin. The same species will be found in the same place although the strain may vary. It is even possible to have two different kinds of *Staphylococcus* in different nostrils! It is not known exactly how one type of bacterium inhibits another, but it is thought that protein chemicals called bacteriocins control or kill other strains of the same species.

It is not easy to give accurate counts of bacteria as they are so small. Studying a normal eco-system the technique is to tag individuals of a given species and then to study their inter-relationships with the rest of their environment. With bacteria this is impossible. The standard tool used by the bacteriologist is the culture-plate, which studies populations, not individuals.

The simplest way of removing bacteria from the skin is to use a sterile pad of velvet which is then pressed on to a culture medium such as a meat broth which is mixed with seaweed agar to form a jelly in the bottom of a flat transparent dish. Each individual or group of bacteria printed by the velvet on to the jelly will grow up within a day or two into a colony of millions of offspring on the agar plate. The appearance of an impression from the face is startling to say the least, and that of the lips enough to deter one from kissing for a considerable time.

Another technique to get a more accurate idea of the numbers of micro-organisms is to press a small cylindrical container on to the skin which is filled with liquid and the skin then scrubbed with a glass rod to stir up the bacteria. This soup is then diluted with a large amount of sterile liquid so that the bacteria are widely separated before it is added to agar plates as before. There is then a good chance that each colony grown will have come from only one original bacterium and a count can be made of the number within the area of the cylinder.

If sellotape is stuck to the skin and then stripped off, it removes a layer of skin scales with their accompanying bacteria, and again the imprint of the tape can be cultured. By repeatedly stripping the same area it can be demonstrated that the bacteria inhabit only the outer layers of the *stratum corneum*, the tough layer of desiccated skin scales, and ten strippings will remove 95 per cent of them. But they also penetrate down the hair follicles and sweat glands where they can only be sampled by cutting out tiny pieces of skin.

The most important factor limiting the number of bacteria in a given area is moisture. If a waterproof bandage is put on the skin of the arm the population rises from its normal level of a few thousand per square centimetre to tens of millions within a day or two. So it is no surprise to find that moist areas like the armpit and groin carry the biggest populations. The figures go something like this (per square centimetre) for a grown man: a million in the armpit, one and a half million on the scalp, 200 000 on the forehead, but only 50 000 per square centimetre on the back and 11 000 on the forearm. These figures are taken from surgically removed pieces of skin, frozen and then sectioned, when a very accurate count can be made.

When there are many follicles and sebaceous glands the deep-living anaerobic bacteria may outnumber the surface ones by a factor of ten.

One puzzle is that some men seem to have bacterial populations dominated by cocci, while others show a preponderance of the diphtheroids which live on fatty nutrients. This is not just a question of which came first, because if the balance is disturbed it returns to favour the previously dominant variety. What is not realized by doctors is that the two types of patient almost certainly react differently to antibiotics because of their different bacterial flora.

The varieties of bacteria present also depend on age. Children have a far more varied flora than adults, and frequently have soil-type bacteria on their skins. Children come into contact with the ground as well as other strange places more often than adults and until puberty their skins lack sebum, reducing the number of diphtheroids. A larger proportion of them also carry *Staphylococcus* in their noses. Old people on the other hand carry a relatively small variety of life, though the decreasing efficiency of their immune system is probably a reason why they are more likely to have yeasts like *Candida albicans* as well as bacteria.

Most people confronted with the fact that they support several thousand million hangers-on have an irresistible urge to have a shower, or even as one reviewer of my TV film put it 'to immerse himself forthwith in a plunge bath full of aviation spirit'. But a bath, with or without detergent soap actually puts *up* the number of bacteria released from our skins by as much as three times for a good ten hours. What probably happens is that the heat and the moisture cause large colonies to break down into smaller ones. That does not sound too bad, but it also means that we shed far more bacteria into the air after taking a bath. Indeed, tests on volunteers who had showered and soaped for ten minutes showed a marked increase in the number of bacteria floating in the surrounding air on their rafts of shed skin as their hosts were dressing.

It is, in fact, almost impossible to sterilize the skin. Even alcohol or iodine only remove a percentage of the surface bacteria, and nothing will penetrate down into the hair follicles and sebaceous glands which will kill the bacteria without harming the skin. This is just as well because our commensal bacteria keep away our enemies. The combination of acidity, dryness and salt, as well as the resident bacteria, make it surprisingly difficult to cause an infection on intact skin. There is only one germ which succeeds frequently, of which we are right to be wary – syphilis.

Some of the bacteria which we can tolerate with equanimity on our skins can be rapidly fatal if they get into the bloodstream. The most celebrated of these 'opportunist' organisms is *Staphylococcus aureus*. Its success as a virulent pathogen is probably due to its ability to colonize rapidly rather than any specially unpleasant toxins that it produces.

A famous example of its effects was the Bundaberg tragedy. It was not long after the introduction of diphtheria inoculations, and the town of Bundaberg in South Queensland had organized a campaign to immunize the local school children. Then on one day in January 1928 twenty-nine children were injected with the anti-toxin. Within twelve hours eighteen were ill, and before two days had passed twelve children had died. The whole of Australia was horrified by the tragedy, and within a week a Royal Commission was established to ascertain what had gone wrong.

The facts soon became clear. A single rubber-capped bottle of mixture had originally been sterile, and had been used the week before to inoculate a number of children successfully. It was then put in a cupboard (in summer in a sub-tropical climate) until the fatal injections were given. Before each injection a hypodermic needle was pushed through the rubber cap to draw up a dose into a syringe. The needle had picked up a few organisms of *Staphylococcus aureus* from the skin of one of the first group of children and had carried them into the supposedly sterile bottle. The wait on the warm shelf gave perfect conditions for the bacteria to multiply to millions of millions; in fact, the bottle should have been visibly turbid by the time it was re-used. Each of the new group of children received tens of thousands of bacteria under his skin.

In theory the tragedy should never have happened. The same needle should never have been used for more than one injection, and the bottle should have been refrigerated and not re-used after the sterile cap was first removed. Still, the severity of the results astonished bacteriologists. Sir Macfarlane Burnet, later to win the Nobel prize for his work on immunology, who led the investigation wrote that the death of over half the children within two days would never have been predicted and pointed to the production of some extremely poisonous substance by the *Staphylococcus*.

It remains an awesome warning of how dangerous the bacteria are which some of us carry quite happily all our lives. Another example is when *Streptococci* which live in our throats are released into the bloodstream by even such a seemingly innocent operation as pulling a tooth. The bacteria can be swept round the circulation until they lodge in the one place where our defensive white blood cells are powerless to get at them: the fibrous tissue of a heart valve. There they remain and grow to a colony slowly and remorselessly eating away the valve until it is destroyed and the man dies, his white cells all the while being whirled past in an impotent flood by the strength of the heart-beat.

Another opportunist bacterium is the *Streptococcus*, which looks like a group of cocci threaded on a string like beads. This has long been dreaded for its capacity to kill off the red cells in the blood, and as the cause of puerperal fever, which before the introduction of elementary antisepsis made childbirth so dangerous. Traditionally it was held that *Streptococci* had their headquarters in the nose, but some recent studies done on Red Indian reservations in America have shown that summer-time *Streptococci* skin infections which commonly result from abrasions and insect bites were transferred by contact from skin to skin of one individual to another. It was known that *Streptococcus* throat infections could cause kidney disease, but now it was found that these apparently trivial skin infections could have the same unpleasant consequences, and in fact were the more likely cause. So far insufficient work has been done to decide how often *Streptococci* form part of the normal skin flora, but the discovery that they inhabit the skin independently of the nose is bound to lead to a new interest in them as they are potentially so dangerous, especially in that hothouse of all infectious agents: the hospital.

When the sulphonamides were succeeded by penicillin and the whole range of antibiotics became available there was a huge surge of optimism amongst medical men. The infectious diseases were done for. Bacteria would never again be a problem with the new magic bullets of drugs. How wrong they were we can see twenty years later. The antibiotics are in retreat and the diseases at best held in check. We are as ignorant of curing virus diseases as we were fifty years ago, and much of the usefulness of antibiotics against bacteria has been squandered.

What happened is a fascinating example of natural selection, which takes place so rapidly with bacteria that it operates from day to day in a hospital ward. *Staphylococcus aureus* is normally very sensitive to penicillin. But in cases where a dose of penicillin has been given to a patient which is only just enough to kill the bulk of the bacteria, a few which are genetically best adapted to resist penicillin will survive. This survival of the fittest ensures that they will go on to breed into the gap left vacant in the eco-system previously inhabited by the killed strain. The penicillin-resistant *Staphylococcus* will soon predominate where penicillin treatment continues. By 1946, 14 per cent of infections in a general hospital were by penicillin-resistant strains, and by 1950 a majority of all *Staphylococcus* infections in British general hospitals were resistant. As fast as new antibiotics were introduced the bacteria developed resistant strains. Nowadays in bacteriology labs in hospitals they use standard test discs, papers impregnated with what were once our best antibiotics, penicillin, tetracycline and streptomycin, to test whether the sample culture of bacteria is still vulnerable to any of them, and frequently it is not. Fortunately not all the dangerous strains of *Staphylococcus* have been equally successful in acquiring immunity to drugs.

Another interesting point is that the bacterium needs to go through two genetic changes to become resistant to penicillin. The first enables it to deal with small doses and the second with large ones. If it was not for the fact that the bacteria multiply in their first resistant form to fill an ecological niche in the hospital, it is very unlikely that the second mutation (against which the numerical odds are extremely high) would have taken place. Similarly it takes a new mutation to acquire immunity to a new antibiotic, and it is only because of the enormous mortality of bacteria in the ordinary way, and the very rapid multiplication of surviving strains that this can happen.

Considering the adaptability of bacteria it is surprising that we are not troubled by more varieties of them. We can only thank the fact that we too have evolved for a long time, and our defences against invading germs have been sharpened in our struggle for survival.

For a long time bacteriologists have tried to establish experimental infections on human skin. As recently as 1965 cultures of a hundred million bacteria per millilitre were applied to skin which had been maltreated in a variety of ways such as blistering, irradiating with ultra-violet, having the surface stripped, or hairs pulled out. Almost all attempts failed, and the skin was thought to have some marvellous self-disinfecting property which quickly killed foreign bacteria. First the acidity of the skin was held to be the reason, but when it was found by experiment that the slight acidity did not make much difference to hostile bacteria, then the fatty acids in sebum were hailed as our protectors. Not until 1971 was it realized that the combination of skin shedding and the inherent dryness of the surface could account for the rapid destruction of applied cultures of germs, provided the normal population of bacteria was intact.

Experiments were carried out to test this theory. They showed that a moisture-proof polythene bandage would moisten the surface and allow an applied culture of *Staphylococcus aureus* bacteria to survive if most of the normal skin bacteria were first removed. This was done by workers from the University of Pennsylvania School of Medicine on 'about 150 male prisoner volunteers, age 25 to 40; most were black. A few were infected more than once.'

Their technique was to clean the skin with alcohol to remove most of the surface population of bacteria before applying a droplet of the *Staphylococcus aureus* culture which was promptly covered with a polythene bandage and left for six days. This produced a red rash within three days followed by an eruption of spots. Interestingly enough, even the presence of the dense colony of *Staphylococcus* numbering millions to the square centimetre did not stop the natural population of bacteria returning, and when the polythene bandage was taken off and the skin was able to dry it returned to normal after about two weeks. This showed that the cocci and diphtheroids of the normal skin are so adapted to skin conditions that they have an ecological advantage even on damaged skin.

Experiments with an organism as dangerous as *Staphylococcus aureus* should not be undertaken lightly. By way of a warning the Pennsylvanian workers point out: 'While we were casting about for an experimental model we placed suspensions on scotch-tape-stripped skin which was then occluded (with polythene). We soon had reason for regret. Within hours the subjects had fever, malaise, pain, and swelling at the inoculation sites,' and the experiment had to be ended with a rapid dose of penicillin.

While such experiments have undoubtedly increased medical knowledge with important potential for future treatment, doubts must remain about the legitimacy of using prisoners in a penitentiary as 'volunteers' for any medical experiments. The pressures on such inmates to make them wish to be considered amenable by those in authority over them are so obvious as to make one extremely sceptical of their true motives in wanting to take part. In Britain such experimentation is not allowed by the Home Office. The appalling possibilities for misuse of a captive experimental population are outlined in the chapter on typhus. If, for convenience or control, the human subjects must be in an institution then there are other communities such as monasteries where an individual's motivation for taking part would be less suspect.

The relationship between skin bacteria and criminals is not confined to the progress of scientific research. The public may benefit rather more directly from a bacteriological forensic technique for distinguishing individuals who have been present at the scene of a crime.

The characteristic microflora of a suspect could become as important to the detective as a finger-print. Or at least this is claimed by Professor M. Gershman of the University of Maine. His thesis is that since the microflora is established shortly after birth and remains comparatively constant throughout life, a microbial sampling of room dust, saliva and so on, might reveal groups of identifiable organisms which would match the pattern of a suspect. There are so many different phage-types of bacteria and the acquisition of these by an individual happens in such a particular manner – from mother, hospital and early contacts – that it is very unlikely that two suspects would support the same organisms. Gershman points out that outbreaks of disease like typhoid can already be traced back to individuals through sophisticated phage-typing methods, and dispersers of *Staphylococcus aureus* of one phage-type can be picked out from amongst many others. It may not be long before bacteria are called for the first time to give evidence in court.

## Yeasts

Another whole group of inhabitants of the human skin are the yeasts and fungi. A yeast is a single-celled fungus which reproduces by budding, in other words a daughter cell grows out from the parent and then breaks free.

By far the most common yeasts on our skins are the genus *Pityrosporum* which belongs to the family Cryptococcaceae. There are two species, of which *Pityrosporum ovale* is at home on most of us. It consists of oval spheres measuring about 2 microns wide and 4 long, and it thrives on our hair and fatty parts of our skin like the scalp and around the nose, where the population can reach half a million per square centimetre.

Once again it is remarkably little studied. There have been claims that there are 155 strains and that 90 per cent of us are carriers; others claim that only 55 per cent of normal males have yeasts. There seems to be an agreement that the more sebum is secreted the higher the yeast population grows, and that it is harmless. There has been a long attempt to prove some association between *Pityrosporum ovale* and dandruff. Seventy-eight per cent of those with dandruff have yeasts, but then a lot of people with dandruff don't have yeasts.

Dandruff appears to be caused both by an excessive scaling and by the scales sticking together to form larger visible clumps. Men, or their womenfolk, appear to be obsessed with their scalps and all that pertains to them. According to an American survey 60 per cent of those who think they have dandruff have only a minimal amount; and only 20 per cent of young men do have the affliction. It decreases in summer, and a normal shampoo will reduce the amount of scaling by 75 per cent after

24 hours, returning to normal by the end of six days. A medicated shampoo containing the anti-microbial agent Selenium sulphide will reduce dandruff permanently to 20 per cent of the former amount if it is used twice a week.

Failure to wash one's hair will not bring on an attack, as was proved in an American prison. Dandruff-prone and non-dandruff convicts were persuaded to wear bathing caps sealed to their heads for three weeks. (Science does not record the comments of their fellow inmates.) Only the dandruff-prone prisoners suffered, and after three weeks they stank.

Dandruff is nothing more sinister than the dried skin scales being shed in clumps rather than individually, and if it was not for the fact that it shows up on shoulders, we would probably ignore it and be none the worse.

But the same cannot be said for *Pityrosporum orbiculare*, a round yeast of about 2 microns in diameter which is thought to be the cause of a scaling condition of the trunk and neck called *Tinea versicolor*. This affects up to 40 per cent of the population of moist tropical countries, no doubt exacerbated by malnutrition and poor hygiene. It is caused when the spherical yeast turns into another form where filaments called hyphae grow into a spreading mycelium or root-like growth of fungus.

Fungi include such widely diverse forms as mushrooms and the nightmarish *Dactylaria* and *Dactyella* which live in the ground and have the power to ensnare tiny worms by swelling up loops of mycelium around them like blood-pressure machines. Fungi spread by means of spores which are extremely long lived and resistant, as anyone who has tried to get rid of dry-rot in a damp house knows. They secrete various enzymes which decompose organic matter and then absorb the decaying solutions.

Just as our skins are proof against the invasion of most bacteria, so they are inhospitable for yeasts and fungi. Again, dryness is a first defence. Then human blood contains a specific anti-fungal chemical, as do tears. In spite of this individuals can carry a wide variety of transient 'visiting' organisms some of which can be unpleasant.

Thrush, the white cobwebby fungus which appears at both ends of the food canal of babies, is caused by the yeast *Candida albicans*. This seems to be part of the normal flora of about 5 per cent of the population, but notably increases in the elderly to about 20 per cent. One study at University College Hospital, London, showed that 3 per cent of babies born there had thrush by six months, and that it was nearly always caused by *Candida albicans*. It can also occur in the bowel and vagina, and is often the cause of unpleasant 'intimate' smells. Sometimes it will colonize the webs of fingers and nails, especially amongst those whose jobs entail constantly wet hands. The fat and diabetic are more susceptible, and it can be fatal to those suffering from deficient immunity.

Damp is also a ruling factor in invasion by the fungi which cause such well-known maladies as athlete's foot and jockstrap itch, although it has been shown that two out of three diagnoses blaming fungal growth are wrong. These conditions, like ringworm, are caused by fungi called Dermatophytes and frequently become invasive when the bacterial population is interfered with by the use of antibiotic creams and large doses of those antibiotics like tetracycline which pass through from the bloodstream to appear on the surface of the skin. Once established these fungi are not easy to remove and are highly infectious (ringworm is frequently caught from domestic pets). The capacity for ringworm to spread is acknowledged in the tradition that no man with ringworm has to remove his hat in the presence of the British monarch.

Perhaps the most serious problem, however, with yeasts and fungi, is the fact that prolonged use of steroids leads to a marked increase in the yeast populations. As many as two-thirds of patients on steroids have been found to have *Pityrosporum orbiculare* which is normally rare. Steroids suppress the body's natural immune defences, as well as having many other therapeutic virtues, but this aspect is often forgotten until too late. Those having massive immuno-suppression, for example for kidney grafts, are even more at risk. One patient at Hammersmith Hospital died of a fungus which normally is confined to lupins.

The sinister potentialities of both yeasts and bacteria should make us all the more grateful for the friendly species whose colonies prevent our enemies gaining a fatal foothold. The least we can do is to try to preserve the conditions which favour our friends. An example of the potential dangers when the skin becomes too wet and poorly cared for is that amongst American troops in the Mekong Delta of Vietnam skin disease accounted for 70 per cent of all man-days lost. During the Vietnam War it was fourth on the list of causes for in-patient hospital treatment of troops, and there were double the number of skin disease out-patients than those for any other condition.

Tests showed that 'Paddy foot' could be produced by immersion in water alone. After three days and nights the water itself produced striking inflammation which allowed the skin to be much more easily infected.

Unfortunately the concept that man is not an island entire to himself but is part of an ecological system has so far failed to influence the man who prescribes treatment. Yet single-minded pursuit of misguided therapy can make things worse, antibiotics may allow an overgrowth of fungi which may not be apparent clinically; fungicides may cause the reverse. The results can be frightening. In the U S Air Force athlete's foot has even been treated by amputating toes.

# 5
# Mites and Ticks

*A good microscope discovers those small moveable specks to be very prettily shap'd insects . . . . The shell, especially that which covers the back, is curiously polisht, so that 'tis easie to see, as in a convex looking glass or foliated Glass-ball, the picture of all the objects round about.*

ROBERT HOOKE

Nothing amongst all the unsuspected secrets of one's skin is more astonishing than the thought that the roots of one's eyelashes are colonized by mites. Few people can confront with equanimity the idea that worm-like creatures which have been likened to eight-legged crocodiles squirm out their diminutive lives in warm oily lairs in our hair follicles.

Since mites, like spiders, have eight legs this means that they are not classified as insects but as arachnids, a class of arthropods or creatures with external skeletons like lobsters or insects. The class called Arachnida also includes scorpions and ticks, and none of them have antennae, but mites and ticks unlike the other members of their class have fused body segments, which gives them a characteristically solid appearance. Indeed Robert Hooke, the first man to make microscopical investigations of them, considered them to be reptiles.

There are claimed to be over a million different species of mites, and in the British Isles alone 1600 species have been classified. They are an extremely successful form of life, and flourish over almost as great a range of conditions of climate as bacteria. They can be both free-living and parasitic, and are adapted to live off the bounty of both plant and animal hosts.

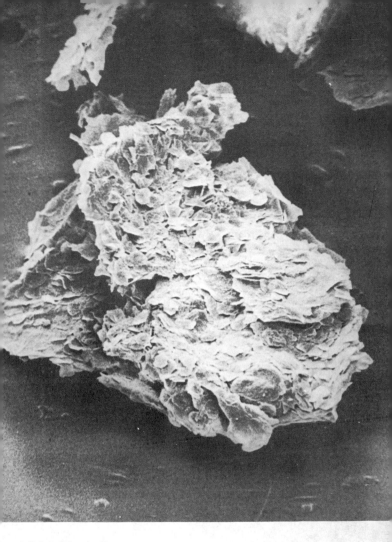

A flake of dandruff.

*Overleaf*

*Top left.* Clean hair ($\times$1000).
*Top right.* Dirty hair ($\times$1000) showing skin scales and sebum.
*Bottom left.* Stubble and a vellus hair on chin, 24 hours after shaving.
*Bottom right.* 24 hours after an electric shave.

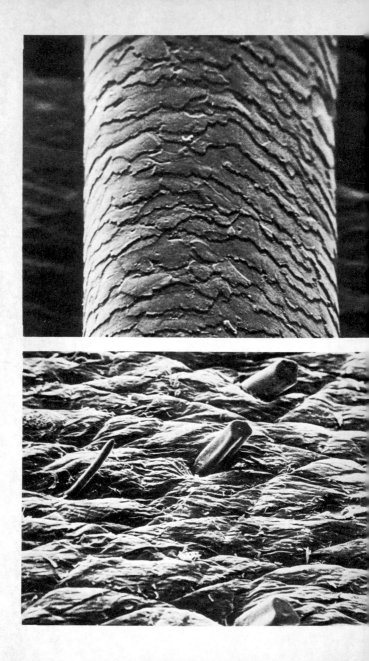

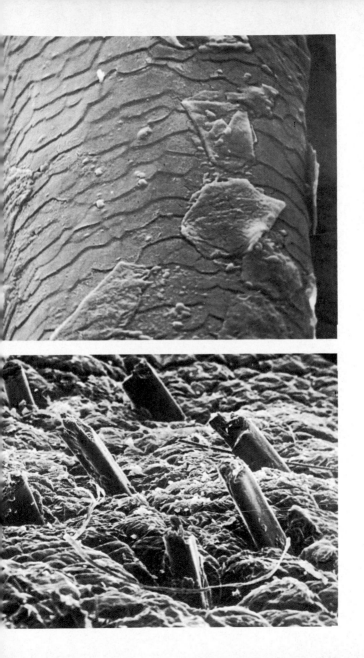

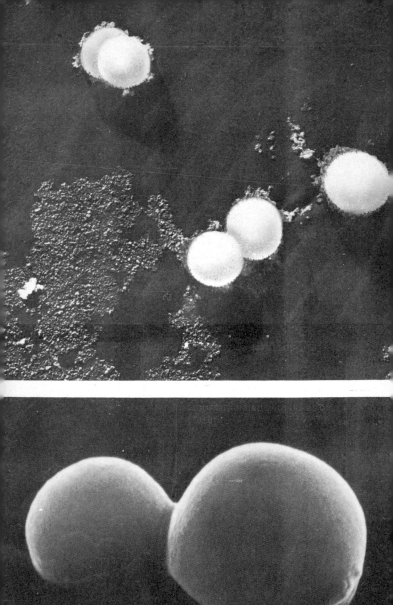

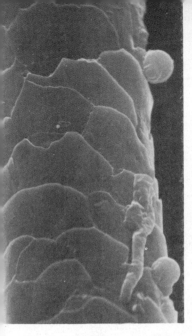

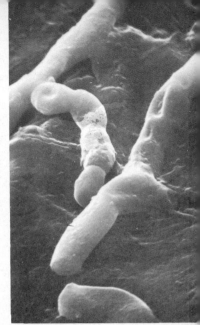

*Above.* Yeasts on hair (×2000).

*Top right.* Hyphae of skin fungi, *Pityrosporum orbiculare* (×8000).

*Right.* Skin fungi (×2500).

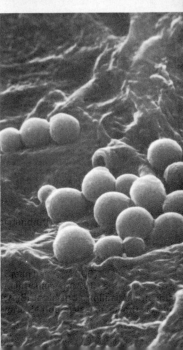

*Facing page*

*Top left.* *Staphylococcus aureus* bacteria (×15000).

*Left.* The yeast, *Candida albicans.*

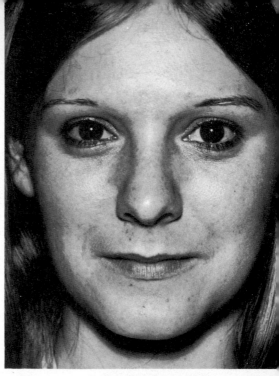

*Above.* Colonies of bacteria from a face print.

*Right.* Colonies of bacteria from hand prints before and after washing.

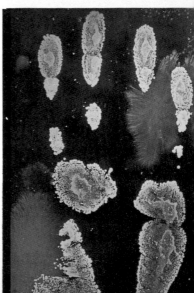

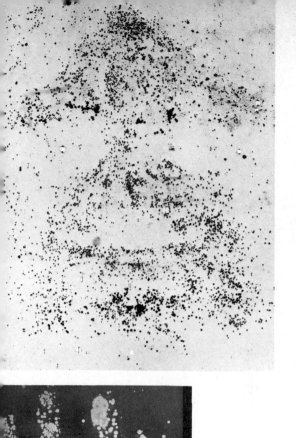

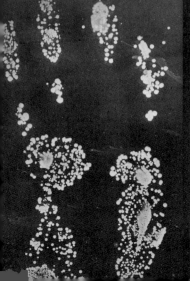

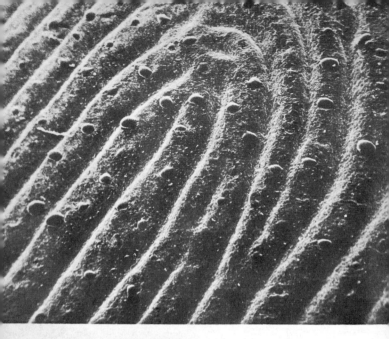

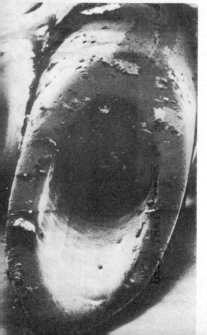

*Above.* Sweat beads on a finger-tip.

*Left.* Electron photomicrograph of a used hypodermic needle contaminated with flakes of skin.

Aristotle called mites *akari* and they are now described as being of the order Acarina. They are impressively tiny, the follicle mite with all its complex anatomy is smaller than the single cell of the human ovum.

The only mite which can be considered our permanent companion through life is the follicle mite *Demodex folliculorum*, which is about a third of a millimetre long with a worm-like shape clearly adapted to help it to crawl in and out of the narrow cavities between the hair and the follicle wall. Until recently their presence was considered to be completely harmless, and quite what effect they do have is still in dispute. However, the related follicle mite in dogs, which appears to be identical although it is unable to live on man, is associated with mange.

It seems extraordinary that the medical profession should have ignored a parasitic mite that lives, literally, beneath their noses, but this was the case until 1967 when a thesis by an American eye-doctor, Tullos Coston, triggered a new fashion for mite hunting. It is not that the mite was unknown, it was first discovered in ear-wax in 1842, and the following year a German published the chilling information that he had found *Demodex folliculorum* in the follicles of the nose of all corpses except those of newborn babies. Coston, being an opthalmologist, was chiefly concerned with their presence in eyelashes (a convenient place to reveal the mite since a lash pulled out will frequently have mites clinging to it). He found that one individual in four had infested eyelids, but other studies which have been done at autopsies where the follicle can be cut open and examined far more rigorously lead to the conclusion that almost every adult harbours the mite on the chin, the nose, or the forehead and scalp. It has even been found in a majority of nipples. All of these are areas supplied with large sebaceous glands.

*Demodices* under the microscope look almost transparent and the pulsating movement of their eight stumpy sucker-like legs is quite obvious. They can cover a distance of 25 millimetres on a dry glass slide in a few minutes, moving the four feet on each side alternately. They can also bend nearly double as if hinged at the centre which doubtless helps manoeuvring between the follicle and the sebaceous gland. The conventional method of studying them is to put them in a drop of olive oil or peanut oil on a slide, when they can be seen to swell up as if gorging themselves on the oil. After about six hours they disintegrate.

The mite apparently always lives head-down in the follicle, gripping the lash or hair with its clawed feet, and the two sexes have developed so that they can copulate in this position. The male has a bi-pronged penis on its back above the second and third pairs of legs, and the female a corresponding vulva on its underside. As many as twenty-five mites have been found clinging to one human eyelash root, and it is difficult to believe that such a high population can be harmless. They are nevertheless well adapted to their environment and a parasitologist who completed a detailed study of their life-cycle found that they developed in the sebaceous gland itself. They are sufficiently small for their individual movements to be below the threshold of sensitivity of the nerves in the skin, so they are not disturbed by any scratching.

The female is fertilized just inside the hair follicle, down which it travels to lay its heart-shaped eggs in the sebaceous gland about twelve hours later. The eggs are about 0·08 millimetres long, they hatch after about sixty hours, and the six-legged larva wanders into the follicle where it moults about forty hours later and becomes an eight-legged protonymph. This nymph has poorly developed legs, so it cannot grip the hair and as it feeds it is carried to the surface of the skin by the flow of sebum. After three days it moults again and forms the deutonymph. After a good feed the deutonymph leaves the hair follicle during the night and crawls around over the skin surface for as long as thirty-six hours before finding another follicle in which it in turn moults after a life of sixty hours to form the adult mite. If a female, it then waits in the mouth of the follicle, but if male it re-emerges to seek out a mate. The total lifespan of the female is about two weeks, that of the male rather less, after which the dead mites tend to block the opening to the follicles, discouraging young mites from entering follicles which are already tenanted. Since the mite is sensitive to low temperatures and also prone to death from desiccation the surface wandering must be a hazardous business.

Quite what the mite feeds on nobody knows. It has been suggested that it might be a secondary consumer, in other words that it grazes on the crop of bacteria living off our skin. If it does, it would play an important part in the ecology of the colonies inside the follicles, but there is no firm evidence that this is the case. Other alternatives are that it simply lives off sebum and other secretions, or that it eats the keratin of skin scales shed from the inside of the follicle wall. *Demodex folliculorum* has strong mouth-parts, that may have been developed to cut a way through the blockage at follicle openings, but recently it has been suggested that the mite may also feed on the lashes or hairs themselves. A heavy infestation of mites leads to 'soggy' lashes which lack the resilience of healthy hair and can easily be removed. Loss of lashes, and now the possibility of some other unusual kinds of baldness may well be the consequence of too many mites.

A large number of mites in a follicle will frequently produce a collar of waxy debris which looks like a clear plastic insulator projecting as much as 2 millimetres from the skin around the lash. This cuffing contains the faeces of the mites and itself may damage the lash.

Another potentially harmful role of *Demodex* is as a carrier of infectious organisms. Mites do not wipe their feet, and must clearly be capable of carrying bacteria and yeasts over quite large distances before inoculating other follicles. For this reason alone it is surprising that they have been neglected by pathologists, whose attitude appears to have been that the mite was unimportant and therefore not worth studying. Since it is only by means of detailed study that its importance can be deduced they cannot be commended for their logic.

According to Dr Coston: 'Many patients have been tranquillized, "eye-dropped", "steroided", and called neurotic, because the ophthalmologist did not think of *Demodex* or know how to find and treat them.'

His own sampling method is to remove four lashes from each

eyelid. These will later regrow. One or two mites per sixteen lashes is a normal sample, but six or more indicates over-population. The patient may complain that his eyelids itch or 'feel full'. Since the mites are averse to bright light they must be persuaded to show their presence by a liberal swabbing with spirit or ether (don't try this near your eyes as they need a local anaesthetic); the mites then quickly back out of the follicles until their tails appear at the lid edge looking like cream-coloured bristles.

It is apparently unwise to tell the patient why the process is being carried out lest 'he feels he must be dirty, and he deeply resents the ophthalmologist's knowledge of their pre-sence . . . . Of course if a haughty or obnoxious attitude is exhibited by the patient prior to their discovery, nothing is more humbling than to announce, "Madame, you have mites." ' A second swabbing with ether a few minutes after the first will kill the mites as they emerge.

The love of *Demodex folliculorum* for sebum means that the simplest way to keep down their numbers is to wash frequently with soap and water. It also means that those who use creams for cleansing instead are laying themselves open to trouble. There is a vicious circle which quickly builds up: the face feels 'dry' so cosmetic creams are used instead of soap for cleansing which increases the growth of the mite which in turn encour-ages follicular scaling and plugging, roughness and itching, which sends the patient to the beauty parlour where the cosmetologist (loathsome word) not surprisingly recommends that lots of expensive cosmetics would be far better than cheap soap. Meanwhile the mites multiply, and can in a heavy infesta-tion number thousands on the face of one individual.

But before the drugs firms rush to make some systemic insecticide which will dispatch them with a single dose, I for one would like someone to find out what relationship they have to the stability of the ecology on our skins. However nasty the pattering of tiny night-time feet on our faces may be aesthetically, it could be that they fulfil a biological necessity maintaining our health.

Far less pleasant to the host are the attentions of the itch mite *Sarcoptes scabiei* whose presence in burrows in the skin causes the characteristic symptoms of generalized itching known as scabies. These can be so intense as to keep the infested patient awake all night. Yet again, in confrontation with this mite the medical profession does not come out with much credit, as can be illustrated by the following true stories.

Recently a young married woman had generalized itching for five months after she adopted a baby with eczema. Two months after the adoption her husband also started to itch. They knew that the baby's mother had had scabies. The baby and the adoptive parents were treated with corticosteroid cream which failed to relieve eczema or itching. The mother was then given steroid tablets with some good result, but she was also referred for a psychiatric opinion. As a result the worthy psychiatrist cast doubt upon the suitability of the couple to be foster parents on account of their condition diagnosed as 'nervous eczema'. All of them had scabies.

During the late 1960s in Iowa an adult mongol man was sent to hospital on five different occasions for treatment of an extensive dermatological disease which appeared as a thick reddish fissured dirty scale. Each time he was taken into hospital cases of scabies soared – in all to fifty-four cases. They included patients with whom he had shared a room, porters, an X-ray technician, and even a dermatologist. The patient was finally found to be covered with myriads of tiny papules. A second look at the skin sample taken sixteen months earlier showed an actual scabies mite beneath his skin. He was swarming with mites.

In 1959 a patient with scabies was exhibited to the San Francisco Dermatological Society as an experiment. The opening speaker suggested the proper diagnosis but half those present maintained the symptoms were not those of scabies.

It is not surprising to discover that in Britain and America there has recently been an epidemic of scabies. The mite is in effect acquiring a social immunity. Medical students are not taught about it and the public believe that if they are clean they will not catch parasites. Doctors don't recognize cases so the disease spreads. A while ago 300 cases were diagnosed in Long Kesh internment camp. To reach such high numbers the symptoms must have been mistaken for some time.

There appears to be a regrettable tendency for doctors to use the strongest weapons left in their chemical armoury whenever they find that a condition does not respond to initial treatment. At present the fashion is to use steroids, which despite their very great value in certain conditions are quite useless in treating parasites. It is particularly horrifying to find how often they are used mistakenly to treat children where they can both retard growth and atrophy glandular function.

The incidence of scabies mites in a population varies in waves as I shall explain later, but in different countries with varying climates and social habits the degree of infestation varies widely. In Tanzania where there are extended families affording plenty of opportunity for infection between adults and children, some villages have been found where every child is infested. Fifty per cent of Bantus in Pretoria have scabies, a recent enormous increase. Forty per cent of five-year-old children in Western Samoa have mites. The Sardinians lead in Europe with 12 per cent of the population infested, and the French have 9 per cent, while in Britain the rate appears to be about 2 per cent.

In Britain the disease is not 'notifiable' – it does not have to be reported to the Medical Officer of Health like other serious infectious diseases – so an epidemic can be well advanced before it is noticed. In the late 1960s there was found to be a major increase in the number of cases treated at St John's Hospital for Diseases of the Skin in London. It was found that the incidence in single young people had risen six-fold in men and four-fold in girls. Historically there have been claims of a relationship between the incidence of scabies and that of venereal disease. But the marked increase in syphilis began in 1956–58 and that of scabies not till 1963—64, and there are signs that the scabies epidemic has already passed its peak. It is still, however, a frequent accompaniment to life in communes.

The human scabies mite is indistiguishable in form from the mite parasitizing dogs and horses and other animals like urban foxes which frequently die from scabetic mange. Like *Demodex* each mite appears to survive only on its true host. *Sarcoptes* can also cause an unpleasant scabetic mange in dogs, and in World War I it was a serious disease of military horses, but the human mite will not survive on either animal.

*Sarcoptes scabiei* variety *hominis* is roughly the shape of some hideously hairy tortoise. It is about 0·4 millimetres long and is just visible to the naked eye. As such it was recognized by ancient naturalists, although it was thought to be the early stage of a body louse and was believed to develop spontaneously from the skin. Aristotle wrote that it could be removed from its burrow in the skin with a needle, and the same method is still used today to demonstrate its presence. It was found to be the cause of scabies as early as 1790. It is in no way competitive with the follicle mite *Demodex* and inhabits hairless areas of skin where the female burrows beneath the surface of the *stratum corneum* usually starting at some natural wrinkle or crevice.

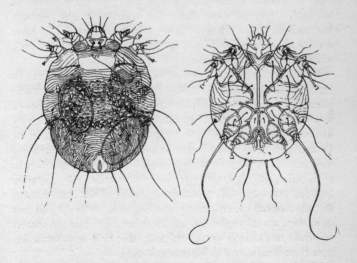

*Scabies mite.* Left, *female;* right, *male underside*

The female mite uses its jaws and front two pairs of legs for digging. These have developed with suckers and a cutting edge on the last joint, so that the mite seems to elbow its way into the skin. Backward-facing spines on the body probably give it a purchase against the tunnel end as it digs, and it burrows at the rate of about 2 millimetres a day. Two or three oval eggs are laid every day leaving up to a total of ten to twenty-five along the length of the burrow which can be seen fairly easily just below the surface of the skin.

The sex organs are arranged in the reverse position to those of *Demodex* with the male organ underneath and that of the female on its back, and to mate the male enters the female's burrow and manoeuvres until they overlap facing in opposite directions. After laying her eggs the female dies at the end of her burrow ending a life of about two months. The eggs hatch after three to four days and a six-legged larva emerges which normally leaves the burrow for the skin surface where it digs a small moulting-pocket. After a life of three days it moults into an eight-legged nymph which, if it is a male, will moult forming the adult. If it is a female it must go through another nymph stage before moulting into the adult form. The whole life history takes from fourteen to seventeen days.

Just how the mite was transmitted from one person to another had been a subject of dispute up to the beginning of World War II. At that time it was keeping two divisions of British troops in hospital at any one time, and there were fears that with the extreme crowding of civilians in air-raid shelters there might be a major epidemic. It was for this reason that a young medical entomologist, Kenneth Mellanby, set up what must rank as one of the most bizarre scientific experiments in history.

At the time, Mellanby believed, as did most other authorities, that infection took place through contact with mites lurking in inanimate objects like blankets, and that the reported increase of scabies was due to soldiers taking the mite home with them on leave. Accordingly he wanted to experiment with volunteers to find out how long the mite could survive in storage in bedding and still be able to infect a new host.

Able-bodied volunteers were scarce in wartime so in December 1940 at the height of the Nazi blitz twelve conscientious objectors found themselves in a house called Fairholme in a suburb of Sheffield waiting to be infected with scabies. Within a few days the public cleansing station in Sheffield had been bombed flat, and Mellanby and his volunteers took over the duties of the scabies squad, getting valuable first-hand experience of the treatment of the condition.

The patients were smeared all over and rubbed well with plenty of soft soap. They were then put into a bath as hot as could be borne and soaked for twenty minutes, after which the body was roughly scrubbed with a brush 'to open the burrows'. Then, after drying, a liberal application of sulphur ointment was made to the body surface and it was well rubbed in. A sufficient surplus of ointment was used to ensure that the underclothes were well impregnated with the medicament.

This crude treatment was surprisingly effective. Just as well perhaps, as few free citizens would go out of their way for a second dose!

At the same time the volunteers were running the domestic matters of the house and the experiments proper soon got under way. Clothing and bedding were brought from a neighbouring barracks, fresh from infected soldiers, and the volunteers either slept naked between the blankets or wore the soldiers' soiled underclothes for a week night and day. Despite this heroic submission to dirty khaki, none of the volunteers became infected. Mellanby explains in his book *Human Guinea Pigs*: 'No one was more surprised than I when weeks and months, covered by a very large number of different experiments of this kind, went by and not one of my volunteers had developed scabies.' Clearly the current views on the transmission of the mite were wrong. The initial nervousness of the conscientious objectors had given way to a feeling that they were frauds and they became very keen to get the disease.

French observations had suggested that the transmission might have a 'venereal origin' and so there were avid discussions as to 'Whether we should try to find some accommodating young woman with scabies to use as a source of infection.' But adultery was not to be performed in the interests of science. In the nick of time the first two infections occurred, following a sojourn in underclothing put on when still warm from the patient. The surprising fact was that the symptoms did not appear until well over a month had passed. This was the first positive clue as to the behaviour of the disease.

Up to that time twenty-five experiments with bedding had had negative results and of thirty-eight submissions to soiled underclothes only two had transmitted the mite. Clearly a more intimate form of contact between individuals was required and it was not long before the 'conchies' found themselves each sharing a bed with an infected soldier. Three out of four of the volunteers were infected in spite of wearing pyjamas.

It became clear that to catch scabies needed close contact with an infected person, and that far from the soldiers taking scabies home the reverse was often the case. Scabies came to be known as a familial disease spread either by sexual promiscuity and perhaps dancing, or by children sharing beds or playing with others. The long incubation period of about six weeks allowed three generations of mites to breed in the new host before any itching or scratching took place, which in turn gave a long infective period before the individual suspected anything. It also frequently disguised the occasion on which the mite was caught. The mite itself was found to be not very hardy; two days in a warm airing cupboard would kill it and the longest survival period was two weeks in a cool damp place.

Mellanby also noticed the differing incidence of scabies in foreign troops stationed in England. Canadians appeared to be far more susceptible than Americans, and he finally came to the conclusion that Canadians as members of the Commonwealth and subjects of the King were invited home to bed by their English girlfriends while the Americans had to make do with less comfortable services in doorways!

The true picture of infection was described in doggerel at a Fairholme Christmas party:

> Recondite research on *Sarcoptes*
> Has revealed that infections begin
> On leave with your wives or your children
> Or when you are living in sin.
> Except in the case of the clergy
> Who accomplish remarkable feats
> And catch scabies and crabs
> From door handles and cabs
> And from blankets and lavatory seats.

In more senses than one scabies is caught by picking up a young adult female, and the Sheffield experiments continued to show the course of the infection, which it was soon found could be mimicked simply by 'inoculating' a volunteer with a fertilized female mite. They showed that after four weeks there was no sensitive reaction but the burrows were clearly visible, after four to six weeks mild itching began increasing in severity, and after six weeks the scabies condition was fully developed.

Regardless of the site where the first mite arrives as an unwanted immigrant it settles in characteristic places. Over 60 per cent burrow in the skin of the wrists or between the fingers, and other favourite haunts are the outside of the elbows, feet and ankles, and male genitalia. Women tend to get burrows on the palms of their hands and young children are highly susceptible on the palms of their hands and feet.

A most important fact in the clinical appearance of the disease is that the parts of the body which itch are *not* necessarily those where the mite is, and the rash which a lengthy infection of a volunteer presented was usually caused by secondary infection caused by bacteria which invaded skin damaged by scratching.

After about three months Mellanby found that there might be a few hundred female mites present, and the volunteers agreed that the itching was barely supportable.

Some kept rough brushes to rub over the skin to relieve the irritation. On cold nights some would rise from a sleepless bed and walk naked through the house, as when the skin was chilled the itching temporarily subsided and sometimes, if sufficiently tired, it was possible to fall asleep before the skin got warm and the irritation returned. Certain volunteers were reduced to sleeping naked as they scratched so vigorously in their sleep that their pyjamas were torn to shreds.

A normal infestation of mites is about a dozen adult females; their multiplication appears to be held in check both by the scratching, the secondary infection, and also the production of fluid as a reaction in the epidermis which floods the burrows. But a patient infected for the second time has no incubation period and at once produces the symptoms of itching, frequently causing the mites to be destroyed before they can gain a hold. Mellanby believes that this is the reason for the wave-like epidemics which recur about every fifteen years. He claims that following a large outbreak a resistant human population builds up and the infestation rate falls until a new susceptible population has been born. But this explanation is disputed by other epidemiologists. It seems likely that epidemics of incorrect diagnosis are equally to blame.

Older people are less sensitive to the attentions of the mite and harbour larger populations, and occasionally there is a case of so-called 'Norwegian scabies' in an individual who has low sensitivity to itching, low immunological response, no secondary infection, and frequently low mental development. In such cases the skin thickens to form a crust which flakes off in plaques riddled with mite burrows. Seen under a lens the activity in these resembles, according to one dermatologist, a crowd coming out of a football match. It has been estimated that such people can harbour over two million mites and they must present a formidable source of infection. With increasing standards of public health such cases are becoming rarer but they are by no means extinct as the Iowa example shows.

In the hope of dealing with high incidences of infection — in some families children are kept from school for years at a stretch as a result of recurrent scabies — Mellanby also experimented with preventive treatment. Perhaps the most extraordinary if not the most effective method he tried was to use a standard sheep-dip, 'having previously determined that immersion for three minutes could be well tolerated by most individuals.'

The Fairholme experiments formed the basis of all future treatment of scabies and probably saved the country a fortune in pointless fumigation of bedding. Dr Mellanby is now better known for his recent role as Director of the Nature Conservancy's experimental station at Monk's Wood, but his interest in burrowing animals has not left him. He is now a leading authority on moles.

Another mite which does not normally live *on* man but which could be said to inhabit his nest is the dust mite, the hairy monster *Dermatophagoides pteronissinus*. To the naked eye it looks like a speck of moving dust against a dark background, and being only a third of a millimetre long it slips easily through the weave of sheets or blankets. It is carried from one house to another on bedding or clothes. It is a scavenger feeding off your shed skin which accumulates in its favourite haunts, the seams and beneath the buttons of your mattress. It likes damp rooms and seldom-used spare beds where the population can run into hundreds. It is discouraged either by the dryness of central heating, or by airing beds which allows the temperature to drop. To most people it causes no trouble, but unfortunately it also gets tossed into the air when beds are made, and the faeces, the moulted cuticles and the mite itself are all frequently inhaled. This causes bouts of frenzied sneezing at bed-making time in some people who are allergic to its presence, particularly in the warm damp days of autumn.

In 1698 Floyer published his *Treatise on Asthma* in which he wrote that 'all asthmatics are offended by the least dust made by the sweeping of a room or the making of a bed,' but the role of the mite was not suspected until 1964.

The first thing that a person does who believes his bed to be

77

inhabited is to sleep in the spare bed, but that too will usually be a home for the mites. Blankets get swapped, clothes are moved from one cupboard to another, beds are given to children, and all serve to spread the population which is impervious to moth-balls and DDT.

The allergic individual can be kept sneeze-free by a rigorous system of elimination of the mite. Mattresses should be covered with plastic and all bedding, curtains, floor-coverings and clothes frequently cleaned, but even then it is very difficult to exterminate all traces of the mite.

It has been found that as many as 40 per cent of people with allergic symptoms are allergic to the dust mite. A simple prick test will confirm if this is the case, and millions of mites are bred to be ground down into preparations for extracts which can be injected as a counter measure. For those of us who have a low sensitivity it may be enough just to vacuum-clean the mattress.

*Dermatophagoides* does sometimes infest the human skin and has been known to burrow into the dermis of the scalp causing small red spots.

Other mites which live off stored food products can be occupational hazards. 'Miller's itch' or 'grain itch' is caused by sensitivity to the grain mite *Pyemotes ventricosus*. A classic out-break of 'grain itch' was in Indiana in 1950 when 1700 visitors to the State Fair had to be treated for as many as 200-300 bites each. The mite infested the straw used in the stalls for the show animals. The same outbreak spread to workers in strawboard factories. Each bite caused a rosy-red weal with a blister.

Stevedores are sometimes exposed to the 'cheese itch' from the mites *Tyrophagus casei* or *T. longior* which thrives in mouldy patches on the rinds of stored cheeses, and other allergic reactions are common enough to have gained popular names such as 'grocer's itch' from poor quality sugar infested with *Glyciphagus domesticus* and 'copra itch' caused by *Tyrophagus putrescentiae*. Most of these are somewhat similar in size and appearance to the scabies or dust mites and have comparable life-cycles.

A survey in Cornwall in 1970 showed that 5 per cent of cases at dermatological clinics were caused by animal parasites. Since patients tend to become petulant and resentful when informed that their pets are infested, it is interesting that in many cases the owner of the animal did not suffer symptoms, but it was the friend or relative frequently visited who did. Owners will often endure a mite rash for years without consulting either a vet or a doctor.

About 1 per cent of all dogs have canine scabies, which can usually be traced back to kennels and breeding establishments. Since there are about five million dogs in Britain it is not surprising that there are records of cases where infestations have spread to human contacts. One consultant at the Royal Veterinary College found that fifty out of sixty-five people who had been in contact with dogs carrying mites had symptoms of mites themselves.

Small dogs kept in the house and handled on the lap were the worst culprits, and the mites would pass through clothing to bite the arms and body.

In dogs the scabies mite prefers the fringe of the pinna of the ears or the hocks and abdomen. The areas affected lose their hair as the disease progresses and become covered with small spots. The inevitable scratching then leads to sores. Handling the ears will, in most cases, produce a scratch reflex which is characteristic of animal scabies.

Cheyletidae are another group of free-living mite parasites undergoing a general increase in Britain, and are found mostly on dogs, but also on cats and rabbits. They can cause an unpleasant disease with intensely inflamed spots which rapidly turn into pustules leading to damage of the skin. The eggs are attached to hairs of the coat where the mite spends its whole life. An infestation causes sensitivity and itching on the back of the animal, or in severe infestations, extensive dandruff and wounds from scratching.

Frequently the nature and source of the symptoms caused by mites caught from animals is misdiagnosed. Instead of the animal host being banished or treated, the human contact is

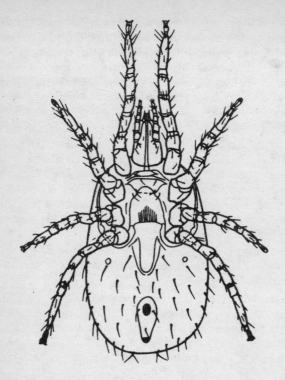

*The northern fowl mite,* Ornithonyssus sylvarium, *underside*

often likely to be treated with tranquillizers, sedatives, antihistamines and psychiatry – while the mite remains unsuspected.

Wild birds can also be the source of trouble. An anxious Minnesota housewife reported to her doctor that she had been scratching compulsively for a week, and when he was unable to find any explanation she returned next day with a pillowcase on which about 100 black dots scurried about with surprising speed. These turned out to be northern fowl mites *(Ornithonyssus sylvarium)* from a robin's nest which was less

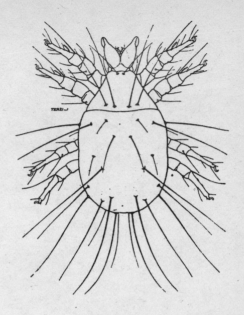

*Tyrophagus putrescens*

than two metres from her bed-head and from which a steady flow of mites covered the window and curtains and bed. Another unfortunate woman was infested and bitten by mites from several bird's nests which had been made in a window-mounted air-conditioner which effectively blew the mites into the bedroom. In neither case was the husband afflicted.

In Britain the most common blood-sucking mite of domestic and wild birds is the red poultry mite, *Dermanyssus gallinae*, and this has frequently been the cause of itching diagnosed as 'persistent scabies'. The important difference is that none of these mites forms burrows like Sarcoptes. Starlings' nests in roofs are often infested with the poultry mite and can be a fre-

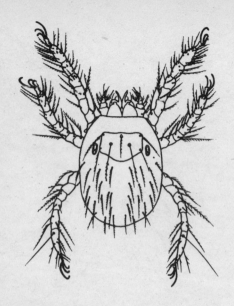

*Larva of the harvest mite,* Neotrombicula autumnalis

quent source of unexplained itching. In birds the mite can carry
relapsing fever, but there are no accounts of this spreading to
man.

A much more frequent annoyance is the harvest mite
*Neotrombicula autumnalis* which is fairly easily recognized by
its figure-of-eight shape, its bright red or orange colour, and its
velvety appearance due to bristles. Its six-legged larva sucks the
blood of man, and it can be very uncomfortable for the
picknicker or amorous couple in the hay who can find
themselves covered in bites causing an intense itching which can
last for days, caused by an allergic reaction to the mite's saliva.
The bites are often mistaken for flea-bites.

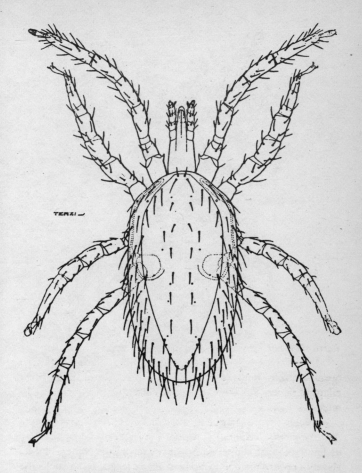

*The tropical fowl mite,* Ornithonyssus bursa

The larvae are small enough easily to pass through clothing and often a line of bites is found at a constriction like that caused by a belt where they cannot climb further. Repellent

83

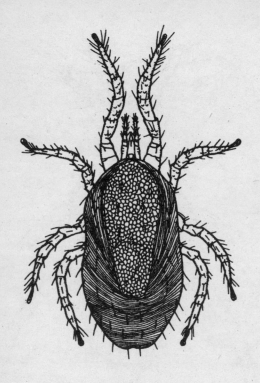

*The most common blood-sucking mite of British birds, the red poultry mite,* Dermanyssus gallinae

smeared on socks and trousers will keep them off. In Europe the mite is no more than an irritant, but there are many parts of the world where *Trombicula* is also a vector of the organism called a *Rickettsia* which causes scrub typhus. An example of this is Tsutsugamushi fever in Japan which exists in a so-called natural reservoir of fieldmice which are bitten by the mite *Trombicula akamushi*. The mite finds its host by a reflex which sends it

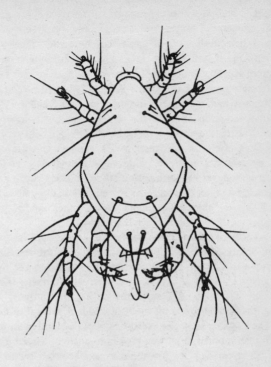

*The male hay itch mite,* Pyemotes ventricosus

scurrying to the top of mounds whenever it senses the presence of carbon dioxide from the exhaled breath of an animal. Sometimes by mistake it bites man. During World War II the retreating Japanese forces left a trail of mites infected with scrub typhus Rickettsiae to attack the pursuing Americans.

In North and South America the equivalent mite is *Eutrombicula alfredugesi,* known as the chigger or red bug.

Ticks are really only large mites, and although there are no ticks which exclusively parasitize man it has recently been recognized that they are vectors for a number of very unpleasant diseases, and as there is so little public knowledge of the risks I am going to include a short section on them here.

The numbers of mites and ticks in the world are almost beyond belief. Studies of the snow-shoe hare and ruffed grouse in North America have led to an estimate of 2·8 million ticks to the square mile, but mites can achieve densities of several million to the square inch. Nature seems to be at her most profligate in the so-called hard ticks; the almost impossible chance that a warm-blooded animal will brush against the precise twig which a tick has chosen to climb is modified by having almost every twig inhabited. Only thus can the species survive, because blood meals are essential to the tick's development. Of hard tick eggs 99.8 per cent never reach the adult stage, and since both a male and female must survive and successfully mate, there need to be a lot of eggs to replace two adults. On the other hand if animal hosts abound the tick population can explode.

An adult hard tick can wait for four to seven years for a meal and has highly developed food reservoirs in its intestines. Since it is sensitive to dry air, it never attempts to climb to the tips of grass stems or twigs in dry, hot weather, which means that the main period for parasitism is the spring or autumn. After feeding, the female drops off the host and lays several thousand eggs. The larva or six-legged seed-tick needs a blood meal within six to fifteen months, and then moults to an eight-legged nymph which again can survive for about a year before a blood meal triggers its moulting into the adult. The female will feed for eight to nine days but the male will only feed for a few hours. Both sexes can wait months for a mate, but make up for such forced abstinence by copulating for as long as a week.

The hard ticks or Ixodidae are so called because of a hard shield on their backs. The Argasidae or soft ticks do not have this dorsal plate; nor are the mouth parts visible from above as is the case with hard ticks.

Soft ticks were put to a sinister purpose as recently as 100 years ago by the Turkmen and Uzbek tribes. They were used for a form of execution in which prisoners were chained to a wall or a bed in a cell into which specially bred ticks were introduced in huge numbers. Since the ticks had been starved first it was a slow and agonizing death.

The best known of the hard ticks in Great Britain is the castor bean tick, *Ixodes ricinus*. Its most important host is the sheep but this tick also feeds on red deer, rabbits, stoats, squirrels, lizards and altogether thirty-nine different species of bird including grouse. The female will swell up on feeding until it looks like a shiny blue pea, and the mouth parts are deeply embedded in the flesh and held in place by spines which makes them very difficult to remove. I vividly remember one occasion when I had been walking in the Highlands of Wester Ross with my wife and we then flew back to London where she disappeared into the airport ladies' room for over an hour. When she finally emerged with a white face she told me that she was covered all over in black ticks which she couldn't get off! For those in a similar plight a soaking in spirit will help to remove them if the head is first pushed towards the flesh to release the spiny mouth-parts. The tick is primarily an inhabitant of rough pasture and moorland grazings, but there are considerable numbers in the New Forest and Thetford Chase.

The sheep tick is the vector for a virus disease of sheep in Scotland and Ireland and cattle in Wales which was first reported 150 years ago. It is called Louping ill from an old Norse word meaning a leap, and is a disease which affects the nervous system paralyzing the shoulder or pelvis. In its extreme form its effect is first to make the animal stray from the flock and then to jump in a curious fashion lifting both hind legs together. As the disease progresses, they begin to shake their heads, turn round in small circles and finally expire. The infection proceeds in cycles of about five or six years, and in a bad year as many as half the sheep in a flock can die. The virus is carried through the different stages of a tick's development, but it is thought that the tick must acquire it from an infected animal. But since *Ixodes* is common to so many hosts it is difficult to trace the full history of the disease.

In man the disease is mild when caught on the moors, and only about a score of infections have been recorded, mostly amongst shepherds, but there have been a few infections where the virus was contracted in the laboratory by research workers in America, and these have had very serious results.

There is an important principle involved here which is bound up with the evolution of the disease. It is not in the interests of a parasite or a disease-causing organism to kill the host, so an organism which produces disease usually implies that the host species has only recently, in evolutionary terms, come into contact with the organism. It is only comparatively recently that sheep have been introduced into Scotland, and it seems likely that the tick and the virus were previously confined to red deer and the small vertebrate animals of the forests.

Viruses carried by ticks come in the group of arboviruses meaning arthropod-borne, and the fact that they can cause serious disease in man was first realized shortly before World War II in Russia, when there were severe seasonal outbreaks of encephalitis (inflammation of the brain leading to paralysis) amongst political prisoners in lumber camps in the Taiga Forest, where the tick *Ixodes persulcatus* abounds. The disease soon became known as Spring-Summer Encephalitis because of the time of the year when it struck, and in its severe paralytic form it has a mortality rate of 25 to 30 per cent and can leave a residual paralysis in survivors. What apparently happened was that the lumber felling disturbed the natural maintenance cycle of the ticks in small forest mammals and birds, and then they transferred to human hosts.

In Western Russia and elsewhere in Europe *Ixodes persulcatus* is replaced by the sheep tick *Ixodes ricinus,* and in the 1950s there was an unpleasant outbreak of a less severe form of encephalitis in Czechoslovakia caused by a virus, which, it was finally discovered, came from goat's milk with which supplies of cow's milk had been adulterated. The virus was then traced back to the sheep tick, and it was found to be present in large numbers of forest birds and animals. It was even suggested that the domestic goats might have been infected by bringing home tick-infested hedgehogs.

Central European tick-borne encephalitis was first isolated in

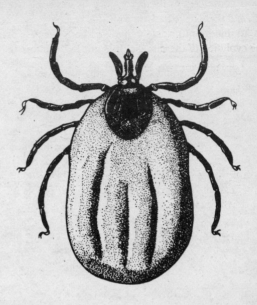

*An engorged female sheep tick,* Ixodes ricinus

Austria in 1927, but it was not until the spreading popularity of camping and rambling brought large numbers of visitors into the forests that large numbers of cases transmitted directly by ticks appeared. In some years as many as 200 cases of the disease occur in Austria, Czechoslovakia and Yugoslavia, and further cases occur in Germany, France, Switzerland and Hungary. These countries could do more to publicize this very real hazard of camping by forests or brushwood where the tick population works out at about one to every square metre, and where up to 1 per cent may carry the virus.

There are several tick-borne diseases such as scrub typhus, 'Q' fever and *fièvre boutonneuse,* but the most severe seems to be that found in the Bitter Root Valley in Montana which acquired an evil reputation in the 1880s when prospectors and settlers found that following tick-bite they were liable to a severe fever. This was fatal in 80 per cent of cases, thus making it one of the most deadly diseases known to man. While working on a vaccine seven US Public Health Service workers contracted the disease and all died.

Rocky Mountain spotted fever is frequently misdiagnosed by doctors in spite of its wide distribution across North America. Although first discovered in the Rocky Mountains, the name is deceptive as it is most common in the Appalachians. It is commonest during the summer, carried in the west by *Dermacentor andersoni* and in the east by *Dermacentor variabilis* and the lone star tick *Amblyomma americanum*. The disease was experimentally transferred by Ricketts to guinea-pigs in 1907 and the organism is called *Rickettsia rickettsi*. In older people it is fatal in 70 per cent of cases, but in younger only 20 per cent. It is not a disease to be trifled with. While most arthropod-borne diseases in the United States are reported to be decreasing, the incidence of Rocky Mountain Spotted Fever has increased sharply in the last decade, from about 200 cases in 1959 to nearly 900 cases in 1976.

The virulence of the disease in Montana has been explained by the fact that an abundance of small mammals live there which might have made the *Rickettsia* more adaptable.

Another disease known as Colorado tick fever appears in a milder form carried by the Rocky Mountain wood tick, *Dermacentor andersoni*, throughout the Rocky Mountains, the Black Hills of South Dakota, and western Canada.

Almost every species of tick yet examined carries viruses or the rather larger Rickettsiae. Many of these are potentially harmful to man. The only safe maxim would appear to be *never let yourself be bitten by a tick*. The simplest way to ensure this is to wear trousers tucked into your socks when you walk in tick country. A liberal application of insecticide on the socks helps.

Since malaria was eliminated from the fens, insect-borne diseases have been discounted in Britain, but it is a safe assumption that they will be with us for a long time yet. For example,

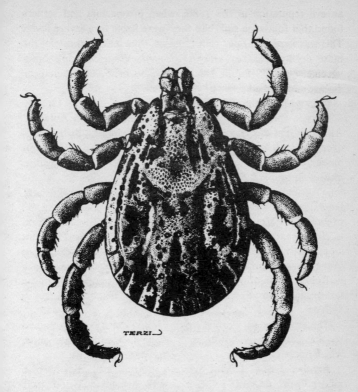

Dermacentor andersoni, *the carrier of Colorado tick fever*

Hayling Island is full of anopheles mosquitoes, and it only needs a visitor to have a malaria relapse for there to be an epidemic. This happened in Northern California in 1952 when a Korean war veteran had a relapse and mosquitoes transferred the malaria plasmodium from his blood to a group of forty school girls camping several hundred yards away.

# 6
# Fleas

*Though they trouble us much, yet they neither stink as Wall Lice doe, nor is it any disgrace to a man to be troubled with them, as it is to be lowsie. They only punish sluggish people, for they will remove farre from cleanli houses.*

THOMAS MOUFFET, 1658

When I was a small boy a generous great-aunt used to provide tickets for Bertram Mills's Circus at Olympia as an annual Christmas treat for myself and all my cousins. In a corner booth outside the big top there was always a rival attraction advertised as 'Positiflea an all live show', a flea circus. One year youthful pleading prevailed against the disapproving frowns of parents and I handed over a warm half-crown and slipped inside.

I remember my disappointment vividly today. There was a ring, and sure enough there were fleas, constrained by twisted girths of copper wire and decorated with incongruous tufts of feather. But the show, as the wretched insects struggled to drag silver chariots or were forced to propel miniature tricycles, struck me as no more than brutality to dumb creatures, a pathetic parody of the fun and noise and excitement of the sawdust ring. The showman recited his patter for the umpteenth time that day in an unenthusiastic monotone and the one moment of fascination was when he rolled up his sleeve at the end of the show and gave his cast a meal on his forearm. 'Wasn't it cruel to harness them with wire?' inquired a sentimental woman. 'Well, think what your own reaction would be if you caught a flea — you would kill it, wouldn't you?' Unimpressed by his question dodging I returned to my parents to manufacture an enthusiastic report to make the half-crown seem well spent.

Twenty years later I found myself interviewing the same showman 'Professor' Len Tomlin for the BBC, and from what I could remember his act had not changed a hop. Only the cast was smaller. Oscar and Oswald still raced chariots at the rate of an inch every few seconds. Pierre and Pedro still scrabbled at pins stuck into bits of cork in a semblance of a sword-fight, Bonzo trundled a tiny roller on a model lawn, and Pooh-Chou the juggler had still been caught in Limehouse on a Chinaman. Business, too, was good when he could open his show, but the supply of fleas was the problem. 'Years ago in my younger days you could see kiddies going to school with flea marks on their necks,' he confided. 'You don't see any of that today.' It was almost impossible to find fleas even when he offered a half-crown each for them.

I have had offers from all over the world to take my show, but you're afraid of one thing, when you get out of the country can you get the fleas? I went to Sweden and I had to send to Majorca in Spain to get fleas every fortnight.

Len Tomlin now runs his show when he can in Manchester's Belle Vue Park, having first opened up his booth on the front at Blackpool in opposition to a German 'Professor' Ronka whom he soon put out of business. He uses only the larger female human flea which lives for about two weeks in captivity if fed every four hours, and relies on his 'Advance Manager' Mr Boulter to find what he calls his 'tiny artistes'. His technique is to go from door to door in what he calls low-classed areas.

I don't mean degrading of people but buildings of age, where people are living pretty rough. Now I always bring a fair amount of cotton wool with me and screw-topped jars. So I have a look around and of course sometimes I just see an odd one or two in a spare room that hasn't been used and I think it's possible there could be more. So I put cotton wool around, tack it around the skirtings, and I leave it there until the morning and nine times out of ten I do pretty well.

Mr Boulter covers hundreds of miles in his quest for fleas, but the vacuum-cleaner now sucks up most larvae before they ever get the chance to mature, and straw mattresses, their favourite haunts, are few and far between. But every now and again a stinking disused mattress reveals a precious horde.

In backward rural countries where fleas are still an expected hazard of daily life they are still treated with something approaching affection. Impertinent nuisances they may be, but not without charm. They are sold in costume as 'Pulgas vestidas' in Mexico, and a group exists in the Museum of Childhood in Edinburgh got up as a wedding party. But the days are gone when in Venice they used to be sold with silver collars round their necks. There are said to be three flea circuses still in France, and others in central Europe, but the famous flea circus at Huber's Museum near Times Square in New York has been closed for a generation.

The scale of past business can be judged from the fact that in the 1830s Signor Bertolotto was able to charge a shilling admission to his 'Extraordinary exhibition of the Industrious fleas' in Regent Street 'Under the Royal Patronage of Princess Augusta', claiming also that many of his performers had been fed by 'Ladies of distinction'. The programme notes survive in the British Museum, and by modern standards it was a lavish affair. A ball with frock-coated gentlemen partnering silk-clad ladies, whilst a twelve-piece orchestra played audible flea-music; the Great Flea Mogul complete with harem, and a 120-gun ship of the line drawn by a single flea. The finale showed Wellington, Napoleon, and Blücher mounted on flea chargers with golden saddles. Well might the heroes have been flea-ridden at Waterloo.

Bertolotto took his trade most seriously and also wrote a book about his performers. In it he relates the end of his oldest flea which died after twenty-three months in harness.

For the last two months it could not leap an inch high, crawling with great difficulty across its little box. As it grew weak I released it from the ten links of gold chain which had been constantly attached to it. It ate voraciously to the last, and was grown to such an incredible size as to be easily mistaken for a bug.

Tomlin has little sentiment to spare on his fleas, and he makes no pretence to be able to train them. 'I get a flea and find out his capabilities. Some will hold things, some will kick them, some will walk, some will jump.' The kickers and jumpers are of limited use, but are still employed for demonstrations. The acts are encouraged by a squeeze betweeen a gigantic finger and thumb or a judicious prod with a pair of tweezers, and the stamina of the insect allows the brutal ringmaster to run as many as fifty ten-minute shows a day.

Fleas, being fairly large, were among the earliest of our parasites to be studied, though it was not until the end of the last century that their enormous importance as disseminators of plague was discovered. Leeuwenhoek's artist rose from the glass with a sigh 'Dear God, what wonders there are in so small a creature', and the flea was soon described by Robert Hooke in 1665 as having a 'Polish'd suit of *sable* Armour, neatly jointed, and beset with multitudes of sharp pinns, shap'd almost like Porcupine's Quills, or bright conical Steel-bodkins.'

There are over 2000 different kinds of fleas, of the order Siphonaptera (siphon without wings). They evolved somewhere back in the Cretaceous Age when insects were the rulers of the earth, and are normally considered to have degenerated in that they are both parasitic in the adult form and have lost the power of flight. Wings are clearly a disadvantage to an insect which wants to move quickly through the dense fur of an animal, and the jump has replaced flight as a means of finding a host. One species of parasitic fly *Carnus haemapterus* does this regularly; it actually sheds its wings after it has flown to a bird host, and then creeps in its new low-profile form between the feathers. It is also worth noticing that feather lice, which have to proceed through feathers which lie on top of each other are flattened from front to back, while fleas which travel between hairs are flattened sideways. Presumably they evolved like this because the fatter ones got stuck and were snapped up by the host.

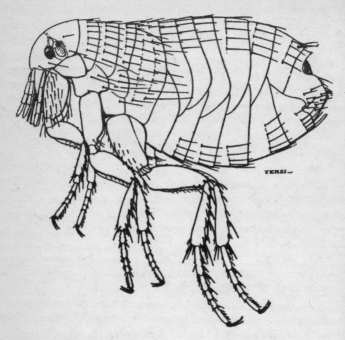

*Female human flea,* Pulex irritans

The human flea *Pulex irritans* has a narrow, rounded head to help it thread its way between the hairs. It has an extremely tough outer covering or cuticle well able to stand up to the rigours imposed by its haphazard method of locomotion. Some species of flea have lost the power of jumping, but they are chiefly those which live in nests which are inhabited so regularly by the host that travel is not important to their survival. A large leap would be a serious disadvantage to a flea living in a squirrel's drey at the top of a tree.

The human flea is equally at home on the badger and the pig, but it is not known which was the original host. One readily acceptable theory is that *Pulex irritans* could only have come to man when he started living in one place, a cave or a hut, since the larva matures on the ground and must develop where there is a good chance for the adult of landing on the host with a casual jump.

The female flea must have a blood meal before it lays fertile eggs. These are nearly spherical and are laid in batches of three to fifteen. From one female 448 eggs have been counted, the large number no doubt compensating for the poor chances of reaching maturity. They hatch after two to twelve days, emerging fastest if the temperature is at an optimum between 17° and 23°C.

The maggot-like larva feeds on organic debris and cannot survive dry heat, which is why centrally heated houses seldom have fleas. It appears to like a trace of sweat or urine and the human flea larva eats refuse such as shed skin scales in bedrooms or dung in outhouses. The rat flea *Xenopsylla cheopis,* however, which is the chief vector for plague, has a larva which has to feed on the blood which is sucked up by the adult flea and squirted out from its anus, so it must always accompany the adult. It is most unusual for an insect to need blood meals in two of its stages of development. The larval stage lasts for one to twenty-four weeks, moulting twice, then it exudes a silky thread, forms a 'U' shape, spins a cocoon and pupates. Its sticky surface ensures a camouflage of dust.

Bertolotto made some strange observations on the larvae:

> If two of these little worms are enclosed in a narrow space, deprived of food, they will attack each other, and each taking hold with its mouth of its adversary's tail, so as to form a ring, will eat one another. This ring becoming smaller and smaller every day for five or six successive days, without either of them leaving their hold, they finally die, and becoming dry are sufficiently hard to be preserved.

In its pupal state the flea can survive almost indefinitely. Long after it is fully developed it can lie dormant until awakening is triggered by vibrations such as the footfall of a host animal. The adult flea quickly emerges and begins to jump in the hope of a meal, but if unlucky it can survive for as long as 100 days.

The way in which a flea finds its host is poorly understood. Experimenters once released 270 marked rabbit fleas in a field of 2000 square yards. After a few days three rabbits put in the field had caught just under half of them, or perhaps one should say the fleas had caught them. In this case the urine of the rabbits appeared to be the attractant. A male flea will approach a female in a series of zigzag jumps as if homing in on a scent, but there is also no doubt that fleas, like some ticks, are sensitive to the presence of carbon dioxide breathed out by animals. The flea also has a sense organ called the sensilium, a saddle-shaped patch on the tail-end of its back equipped with long thin bristles connected to nerves beneath the cuticle. It seems that these detect air currents, though how this would help the flea to find its host is not clear. Even stranger is the flea's ability to recognize X-rays. If one is put in a beam it will speedily hop away.

While a flea is feeding it stands on its middle and back pairs of legs, and with its head down sometimes folds the front pair upwards over its body. Two pairs of palps feel the skin surface of the host and then two lance-like blades each equipped with four rows of teeth jab a hole. Saliva is injected to stop the blood clotting and then a third blade is squeezed up against the two others to form a triangular cross-section tube up which the blood is sucked. The tropical rat flea, *Xenopsylla cheopis,* which also bites man, will imbibe many times its own weight in blood which passes through a special organ in the inside of its crop, formed of a group of inward-pointing spines. This serves to break up the blood corpuscles of the host, but it also plays a crucial role in the dissemination of plague. If the flea feeds on an animal invaded by the plague bacterium, the bacteria become fixed on these spines, and as they breed very quickly inside the flea's midgut they form a plug. The flea cannot get more food into its gut, so it tries again and again puncturing the skin of other hosts, each time regurgitating bacteria into the wound. It is small comfort for the human victim to know that the disease is often also fatal to the flea.

The characteristic bites of a flea, arranged in groups with a central puncture-mark clearly visible, are well known, and can produce acute discomfort. A weal is produced, which can be as big as a walnut, by the irritation of the flea's saliva. Some individuals become allergic to flea-bites and can become seriously ill, but there is relief available for them now in the form of an extract of ground-up rat, cat or dog fleas which can be injected to desensitize them. The effect on the tissues beneath the skin is caused chiefly by histamine. After a 'bite' or puncture of the skin-cells the blood capillaries open up to allow increased blood-flow and at the same time they become more permeable allowing fluid from the blood to seep into the tissues to cause the pallid weal surrounding the bite. The enlarged capillaries also account for the red flush around the area owing to the increased blood-flow which remains some time after the weal has been absorbed into the blood.

The study of the flea was for a long time held up to ridicule as a fatuous activity for a man. Aristophanes in his comedy, *The Clouds,* parodied the teachings of Socrates by making out that the master deduced the length of a flea's leap by making a wax impression of its foot. But man's destiny is now known to have been so influenced by the flea, which in the Middle Ages killed a quarter of the population of Europe, that flea physiology is now taken in deadly earnest. There is little doubt that the world expert on fleas is Dr Miriam Rothschild who keeps a microscope in her bedroom in a manor house near Oxford, and works on her beautifully stained sections of fleas until she falls asleep at night. The following paragraph is from the book she wrote jointly with Dr Theresa Clay, *Fleas, Flukes and Cuckoos*:

Human beings are apt to regard their own personal structure as 'normal' and everything that differs from it as distinctly humorous. It is difficult for them to realize that fleas breathe through holes in their sides, have a nerve cord below their stomachs and a heart in their backs, or that certain other arthropods lay eggs through their elbows, urinate through their heads and regularly practise virgin birth.

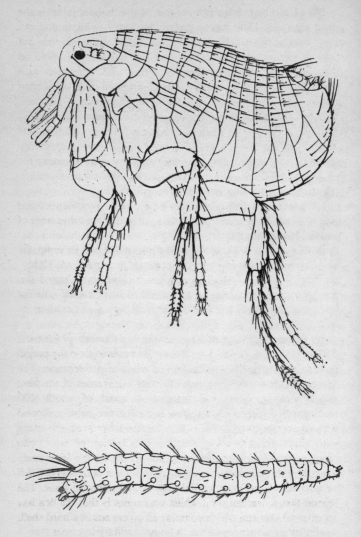

*Male rat flea and larva,* Xenopsylla cheopis

But of all the remarkable aspects of the flea, its jump is the most engaging. Fleas have a natural tendency to climb and can even walk up a vertical sheet of glass if the surface is wet, but they rely on jumping for escape and also to gain a foothold on their host. The human flea can jump about 20 centimetres high and about 150 times its own length, the equivalent of a man clearing a quarter of a mile from a standing start. Of course, fleas have scale on their side. The prodigious feats of flea-power are due to the fact that the volume and mass of an animal depend on the cube of its linear dimension, while the energy developed in a muscle depends on its cross-sectional area or the square of the dimension. The smaller the body of an animal is, the stronger in relative terms is its muscle power.

But small size produces disadvantages too. When an animal jumps it accelerates itself upwards by a springing movement of its legs. It can only accelerate while its legs are straightening, but both flea and man have to reach the same speed to jump the same height, even though a flea weighs only an eighty-thousandth of an ounce. This means that the short-legged flea has to undergo a colossal acceleration to launch itself into the air, especially because it jumps from its knees rather than its feet.

By filming the jump of a rat flea with a camera which took 3500 frames in a second Kim Parker was able to time the period of acceleration which in turn gave the rate of acceleration. The flea clears the foothold in about four or five frames of the film, which means that it has reached a speed of about 100 centimetres a second in less than two thousandths of a second with an acceleration of 140 g. So a flea launches itself into space with about about twenty times the acceleration of an Apollo moon rocket. Put in another way, the forces on the flea's body caused by this acceleration are equal to what a man would feel if he crashed his car into a solid wall at 200 miles an hour. The reason that a flea can do it whilst we cannot is that the flea has an external skeleton which contains all its organs in a hard shell. In similar circumstances a man's body would fly to pieces.

Not only can the flea jump in this remarkable way with

impunity, it can also bounce off solid objects without coming to harm, and the deceleration is then likely to be a great deal larger than the initial take-off rate. As a flea jumps it tumbles through the air and it cocks its front pair of legs over its head so that whichever way up it bounces on the host it is ready to grab its hair.

The very rapid acceleration for the jump cannot be produced by ordinary muscle, so the flea has developed a sort of spring of a protein called resilin which is compressed by powerful muscles to store energy which can then be released suddenly by a type of trigger to project the insect into the air.

The flea is not alone in using resilin. The click beetle flips itself into the air with the same substance with even greater vigour, and has been measured accelerating at 380 g. At the same time its brain is subjected to an acceleration of about 2000 g. which it apparently survives without even a headache.

The larger the host animal the flea parasitizes, the larger the flea's jump must be, and the more resilin it needs. So far the largest lump of resilin that Dr Miriam Rothschild has found is in the leg of a flea which lives in the nostrils of an Indian deer.

Surprisingly the largest British flea, 5–6 millimetres long, lives on moles and the smallest British mammal, the pigmy shrew. To the same scale the equivalent would be to have a small predatory lobster inside one's clothes.

It is difficult for most of us now to appreciate quite how common fleas were in comparatively recent times. They have been the scourge of the traveller since time immemorial. Nor were they confined to the Old World. California had an unenviable reputation for fleas and the early missionaries found that they could not make the Red Indians change the construction of their simple huts because they preferred to set fire to them when the fleas became too insistent and then build another which only took two hours.

One later visitor to a ranch near the site of Redwood City found that his white socks were covered with 'pepper in motion'. The owner then told him that the family routine for sleep was to take off all their clothes, leave them on the floor and make a dash up a stick ladder to a high attic where they slept. A similar evasive technique had been reported by Marco Polo who wrote that Indian nobles hoisted their beds to the ceiling with pulleys to get out of range.

In the nineteenth century the cockney slang for a brothel was a 'flea and louse' being also a rhyme with disorderly house, and a sailor might well talk of a night 'catching fleas' with ladies of easy virtue. Seafaring stories frequently allude to flea-ridden islets at which the locals will not land, where a footfall awakens a ravenous horde of pupae.

The vacuum-cleaner has proved so effective in sucking up flea larvae and living conditions have become so much drier that the human flea is vanishing, but there are still houses in London infested with fleas. Camden is a borough which sports a particularly tough variety according to the pest control officers, and the passenger ferries to Ireland are notorious, but most human flea-bites are now caused by cat and dog fleas, which are equally at home on either animal or man. The cat flea, *Ctenocephalides felis,* likes dry conditions, and the abundance of fitted carpets ensures a ready-made nature reserve for their multiplication. The vacuum-cleaner can never get at the last 25 millimetres of fabric next to the skirting or the radiator where the cat likes to sit and where the flea larvae incubate. Cats can harbour scores of fleas; one keen entomologist once collected a spoonful of flea eggs like fine sugar, from the lap of a visitor who during tea was affectionately fondling his kitten.

Because the cat flea is so small it is frequently unsuspected as the cause of a rash. A typical example was a boy of seven in Newcastle who had a spotty rash ever since he was a year old. Finally it was noticed that his grandmother sat in a rocking-chair all day in the warm kitchen and the family cat used the same chair at night. Old people either do not get bitten so much or do not respond with weals to the bites, so Granny's function as an incubator was not suspected. When at last the rocking-chair and cat were dosed with insecticide the child had relief for the first time in six years.

The dog flea, *Ctenocephalides canis,* is equally partial to a

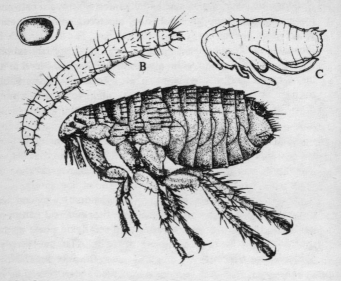

*Cat flea; A: egg; B: larva; C: pupa*

human feast, and one survey of 2000 fleas collected from humans in England revealed that half of them were dog fleas.

Fleas appear to prefer women to men if given the chance; one in a double-bed usually ends up on the wife, a source of marital strife remarked on by Linnaeus. But there also seems to be some factor which will attract fleas to one individual rather than another. In search of experimental evidence a German entomologist, Karl von Frisch, once paraded up and down the bedroom of a flea-infested hotel in Naples in his nightgown with a colleague in similar attire. Von Frisch bagged an average of five fleas and his companion thirty to forty, but it was von Frisch who suffered from large red blisters from the bites while his companion reacted hardly at all.

It seems likely that hormones are responsible for the attraction of the female to the flea, and the rabbit flea provides a

104

remarkable example of how their influence can work. *Spilopsyllus cuniculi* also accidentally infests farmyard cats and frequently shows up as black dots clustered round the ears where they cannot easily be groomed out. The female flea is incapable of breeding unless it is feeding on a pregnant rabbit, and ten days before the rabbit gives birth the hormone level in its blood starts the flea's ovulation. Then by the most remarkable timing the moment the young rabbits are born the flea runs down the mother's nose and on to the baby rabbit as it is being licked clean by the mother. When the fleas feed on the baby rabbit they become sexually attractive to their partners, they mate, and several days later lay eggs. This synchronization of generations ensures that the fleas parasitize each generation of rabbits and so become widespread in the rabbit population.

Leeuwenhoek's discovery of a mite parasitic on a pigeon flea inspired Dean Swift's immortal lines on the universal nature of parasites, though he was referring to plagiarizing poets at the time, but there are various species of the mite family Tryoglyphidae which have adopted a method of passive dispersal in the nymph stage. The egg hatches normally into a six-legged larva which develops into an eight-legged nymph, but after moulting again it turns into a form called the hypopus which has suckers on its belly which are used to attach itself to some other insect in order to hitch-hike to a new home, a method of dispersal called phoresy.

Another much more specialized species of flea parasitic on man is the chigoe or sand flea, *Tunga penetrans* (not to be confused with the chigger, certain larval mites). The chigoe seems to have developed in South America from where it spread to the West Indies and Africa. The early stages of its development are similar to those of *Pulex irritans,* the egg develops on sandy soil and hatches after about two weeks to form larval nymph and pupa reaching the adult stage after seven to ten days. The female then seeks out a host which may be a rat, mouse, chicken, pig or man where it burrows into the skin between the toes or under the toe-nails. It mates *in situ* and produces thousands of eggs swelling its body to the size of a pea producing an intense itching. The eggs are then scattered back on to the ground and the female dies. It is possible to remove the flea complete with eggs intact on the end of a pin, but if left in place it will cause a hard red bump with a black dot in the centre which is the tail-end of the insect through which it defecates and lays the eggs. Frequently the skin suppurates and develops a pustule which can become infected by bacteria leading to the loss of toes frequently seen in West Africa.

There is an account by Walton in his history of Hispaniola of a Capuchin friar who in the interests of scientific study permitted a colony of chigoes to become established in one of his feet 'but unfortunately for himself, and for science, the foot entrusted with the precious deposit mortified, was obliged to be amputated, and with all its inhabitants committed to the waves.'

Even more unpleasant are the cases where tetanus gains a foothold in the wound made by the flea, as in Costa Rica where there were 250 deaths recorded in four years in the early fifties.

The chigoe can be avoided simply by wearing shoes, but without them very large infestations can quickly develop. One man who was lost for some days in a sandy region was found to have 150 embedded in his feet.

# 7
# Plague

*Death came driving after, and all to dust dashed Kings and Knights, Kaisers and Popes, learned and lewd, he let no man stand even, that ever stirred after. Many a lovely lady, and lemans of Knights, swooned and swelted for sorrow of Death's dints.*

FOURTEENTH-CENTURY CHRONICLE

The connection between fleas and plague was not made until the 1890s, by which time the number of known species of fleas had risen from the two recorded by Linnaeus to about seventy. In 1894 in Hong Kong the Japanese bacteriologist Kitasato discovered the plague bacillus and another Japanese scientist Ogata in 1898 first outlined the role of fleas as a vector. This was confirmed independently the following year by the Frenchman Simond, but it was not until 1903 that the amateur naturalist Charles Rothschild, who pioneered the study of fleas in England and founded the flea museum formerly at Tring, discovered the most potent vector of the plague *Xenopsylla cheopis Rothschild,* the tropical rat flea. He named it from the pyramid of Cheops in Egypt where it was found. Charles Rothschild, Dr Miriam Rothschild's father, was a remarkable figure who bought an estate at Ashton near Oundle because he found there the rare butterfly, the Chequered Skipper. Later he built a model village there with a pub named after the butterfly.

It is odd to associate the eccentric passion for animals of this wealthy aristocrat with the saving of millions of lives from a horrible death, but it is sufficient to record the scepticism which met the key discoveries of flea transmission of plague to understand just how important these discoveries were.

In the 1890s a great pandemic of plague was sweeping across Asia, it reached Hong Kong from Canton in 1894 and then was carried by sea to Bombay. By 1903 a million people a year were dying from plague in India alone and the disease had spread to Java, Japan, Asia Minor, South Africa, to the shores of North and South America, and to Portugal, Austria, and European Russia.

The British Plague Commission was based in Bombay, and they refused at first to accept the evidence that the disease was carried from rat to man by fleas. Their experiments disproved it, and only later did they find that they were using the wrong species of flea. The human flea is only rarely capable of transmitting the plague, and the concentration of plague organisms seldom reaches a high enough level in human blood to be transferred by the human flea from one individual to another. But Australia was menaced from Bombay, and research was concentrated in Sydney where the role of the flea was firmly established in 1910. By then the threat had passed, but not without a terrible loss of life which some estimates put as high as a hundred million lives, including ten million Indians. With such figures the ravages of infectious disease dwarf the campaigns of even the most bloodthirsty generals.

The relationship of plague to rats had been noted as early as 1568 in Scotland where it was considered a sure sign of plague to see rats, moles, and other underground creatures forsaking their holes. In the 1850s the high mortality of rats was noted in India as a portent of plague, and in 1878 a French missionary to China wrote:

The approach of bubo-plague may often be known from the extraordinary behaviour of the rats, who leave their holes and crevices and issue on to the floors without a trace of their accustomed timidity, springing continually upwards from their hind legs as if they were trying to jump out of something. The rats fall dead, and then comes the turn of the poultry, pigs, etc.

The wisest men of the age were so ignorant of the process of disease that the conclusion of the time was that plague must be a 'pestilential emanation slowly rising in an equable stratum from the ground the smallest creatures being first engulphed.'

Plague was known to have a traditional focus in Egypt and it was held to be caused by the heat, the water in the soil from the Nile floods, and the rapid putrefaction of bodies.

Charles Creighton, an anatomy professor at Cambridge University wrote a history of epidemics published in 1891, and came to the conclusion that plague was the result of poorly buried corpses, 'a soil-poison having a special affinity to the products of cadaveric decomposition' from which premise he accounted for the fact that clergy had proved to be highly susceptible to plague outbreaks in Britain! It seems incredible that such beliefs should hold currency twenty years after Koch had demonstrated that anthrax was caused by a bacillus.

Now it is known from observation that during an outbreak in rats (an epizootic) fleas leave the decimated rat population to find their food on normally less favoured hosts such as domestic fowls, mammals and man. *Yersinia pestis,* the plague bacillus, is chiefly a parasite of rats, and human infections are only an accidental consequence of an outbreak amongst rodents. The bacillus is a gram negative, rod-shaped bacterium which also appears in snake-like, rounded, and globular forms, and a bite from the rat flea which has had its gut blocked by the bacteria may result in the injection of 25 000–100 000 bacilli beneath the skin.

This is frequently too large an inoculation to be effectively combated by man's immune system and the bacilli multiply in the nearest lymph glands, usually in the groin or armpit, causing a high fever. After an incubation period of two to five days a painful lump develops known as the bubo, formed by the swelling of the lymph gland which drains the bitten area. This is usually livid red or purplish and may swell to the size of an orange causing intense pain before breaking and suppurating. The mortality without treatment is about 80 per cent. Death occurs usually within five days.

The bacillus can also spread throughout the bloodstream when it is known as septicaemic plague and is characterized by haemorrhages under the skin, dark purple blotches of blood which gave rise to the name Black Death, whose victims die 'in a rage of fever', frenzy and delirium within a few hours. Another form is pneumonic plague caused by infected blood passing to the lungs causing pneumonia. The sputum becomes stained bright red with blood and the bacillus can be transferred to dozens of others by droplet infection, particularly in crowded conditions. It is also rapidly fatal, and is said to be the most deadly disease from which man suffers.

Plague is still with us. It still appears annually in some areas of Africa, Latin America, and the Far East, and indeed one of the greatest puzzles to scientists studying epidemics is why we have not had other great outbreaks in recent times. In 1966 there were over a thousand cases confirmed by laboratory tests and 134 deaths. In the same year in Vietnam there were over 500 deaths reported as being from plague, so we should look at past epidemics with the knowledge that it could happen again, in spite of the effectiveness of antibiotics, in areas where modern medication is not available.

One of the earliest references to plague is in the Bible which reports how plague smote the Philistines in 1320 BC for stealing the Ark of the Covenant (1 Samuel 5-6 and 1 Kings 5) but the earliest on which there is detailed information is the plague of Justinian which broke out in Egypt in AD 540 and in two years reached Byzantium where it was soon causing 10 000 deaths a day. 'Finally there was a scarcity of graveyards, the roofs were removed from the towers of the fortifications, the interiors filled with corpses and the roofs replaced.' The plague spread throughout the entire Roman empire. It lasted for three generations and Gibbon concedes that a hundred million people may have died as a result. It was almost certainly a major factor in the fall of the Roman empire. And a hundred million then represented a far greater proportion of the population than the same figure did in the 1890s.

As Gibbon relates:

The triple scourge of war, pestilence and famine afflicted the subjects of Justinian, and his reign is disgraced by a visible decrease of the human species which has never been regained in some of the fairest countries of the globe.

The next great pandemic to sweep Europe is said to have begun in 1346 when a settlement of Italian merchants was besieged for three years at Caffa, a small fortified town on the Crimean straits. Plague amongst the besieging Tartars was killing thousands, and turning to every aid to bring about the rapid surrender of the town, they catapulted the corpses of their dead over the walls. But the siege was relieved and a shipful of Italians escaped and made their way to Genoa. Within days of their arrival the Black Death began. In three years a quarter of the entire population of Europe was dead and the numbers in England and Italy were halved.

The Black Death reached England at the port of Weymouth in early August 1348 when the country was still rejoicing in the triumph of the battle of Crécy and the capture of Calais. Soon it had spread to Bristol and in spite of efforts to contain the outbreak by closing the Bristol roads, Gloucester was infected next. From there it reached Oxford and from Oxford the plague came to London where Parliament was prorogued on 1 January. By the spring it was at its height attacking men rather than women and mostly the young and strong while the aged and infirm were spared. Two hundred bodies were buried in one day in a single London cemetery while in the villages only the women and children were left alive to till the land.

A law to keep prices and incomes at the 1346 level could do nothing in the face of the lack of men to reap the harvest, and that summer a reaper could earn eightpence a day and his food, while there was such a surplus of produce that a fat sheep would only fetch fourpence and a cow a shilling. In vain did the lords of the manor try to keep their bondsmen in their control, and the whole social order cracked under the scarcity of labour. Across Europe 200 000 villages were completely deserted, and the bondsmen fled across the empty countryside to the freedom of the towns.

Petrarch describes the Black Death in Italy and the vast and dreadful solitude over the whole land:

> If you inquire of historians they are silent; if you consult the physicians they are at their wits' end; if you question the philosophers they shrug their shoulders, wrinkle their brows, and lay a finger on their lips. Is it possible that posterity can believe these things? For we who have seen them can hardly believe them.

The plague returned four more times in the fourteenth century attacking those who had escaped the first epidemics and the children who had been born since. In 1361 the *pestis puerorum* struck chiefly at the children of the upper classes. The frantic parents would bar their windows and fumigate their rooms with bay leaves, juniper, and borage, sprinkling the stone flags with water of vinegar and roses; but the plague swept on.

Had the plague remained in England it is likely that subjected to repeated attacks the population would have become largely resistant by the process of survival of the fittest, and a low level of relatively harmless infection would have remained. But depending as it did on a prior plague in rats, which was only viable when their numbers had increased to a certain critical level, it came rarely and so with undiminished fury. There were repeated plagues in the Tudor period. Henry VIII moved his court to Hampton which he approached by river to avoid contamination on the road. And from his reign dates the first surviving plague order:

> Set the sign of the cross on every house afflicted for forty days ... no sick person to go abroad for one month ... kill dogs other than hounds, spaniels or mastiffs and confine those.

Cardinal Wolsey carried with him everywhere an orange 'filled with a sponge of vinegar or other confection against pestilential airs', and in 1563 20 000 died in London – a sixth of the population.

In 1603, the last year of Queen Elizabeth I's reign, the toll in

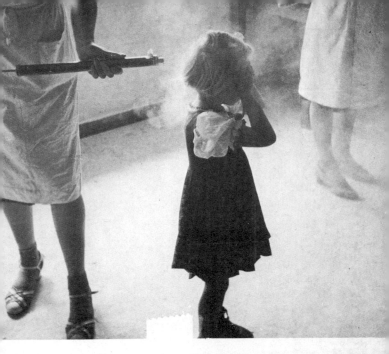

*Above,* De-lousing with D.D.T.
UNICEF, 1945.

*Right.* The female head louse,
*Pediculus humanus capitis.*

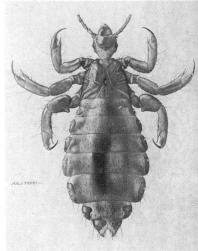

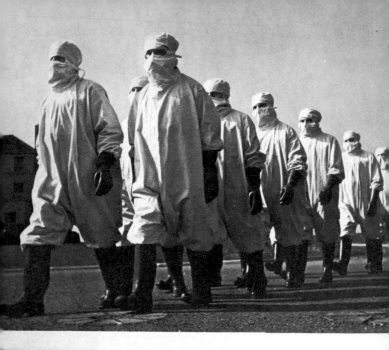

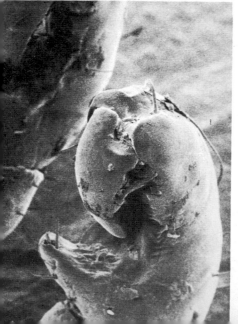

*Above.* An anti-typhus squad goes into action, London 1942.

*Left.* The claws of a crab louse.

*Facing page*

*Top.* Human flea from Robert Hooke's Micrographia.

*Bottom left.* The human flea, *Pulex irritans.* (*Crown copyright*)

*Bottom right.* The head of a human flea. (*Crown copyright*)

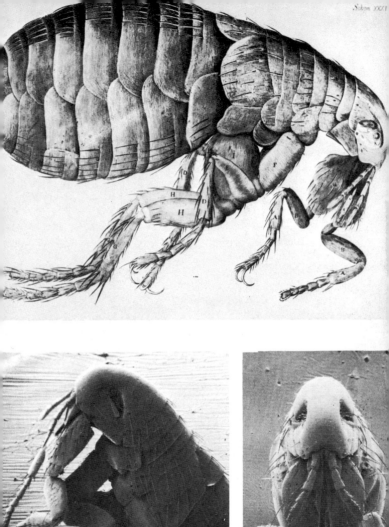

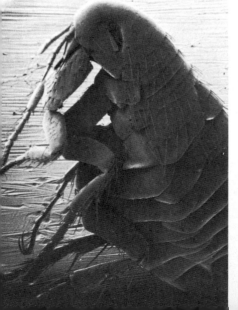

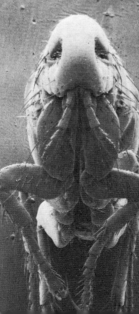

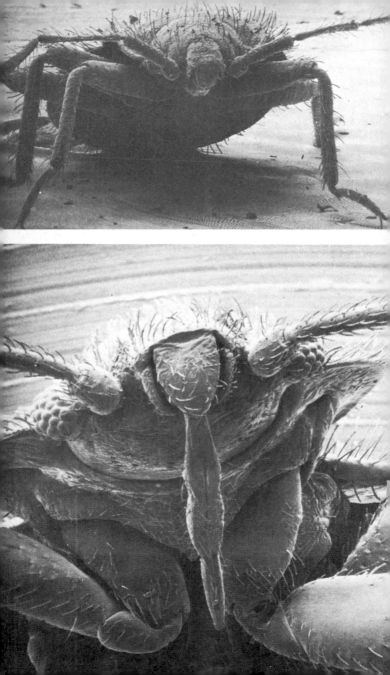

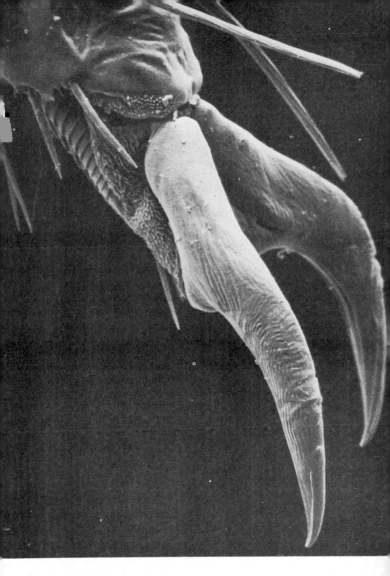

*Above.* A close-up of the claw of a bed bug. (*Crown copyright*)

*Top left.* The adult bed bug. *Cimex lectularius* (*Crown copyright*)
*Left.* The bed bug's proboscis (×90) contains stylets to lance skin. (*Crown copyright*)

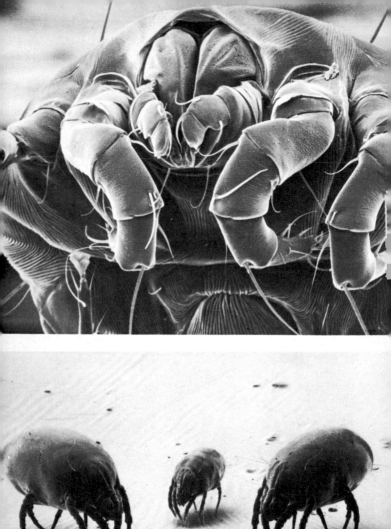

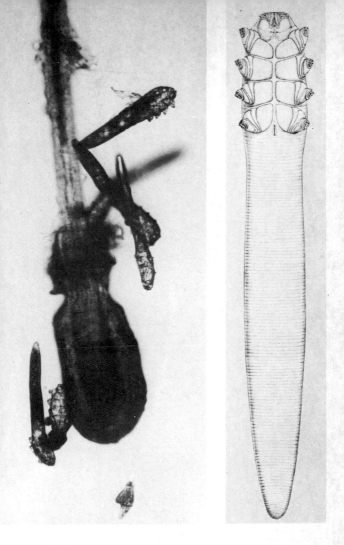

*Above left. Demodices,* the follicle mite, and a lash root.

*Above right.* The underside of the female follicle mite.

*Top left.* A close-up of the front legs and jaws of the house dust mite, *Dermatophagoides pteronissinus.*

*Left.* House dust mites and a flake of their diet, human skin. (*Crown copyright*)

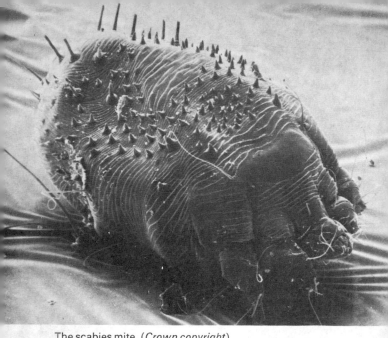

The scabies mite. (*Crown copyright*)
A scabies mite in its burrow in the human skin. (*Crown Copyright*)

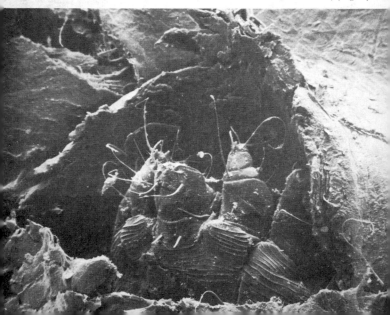

London rose still higher to 30 000 dead. The Queen moved to Windsor Castle and had a gallows set up to hang all those who tried to follow her example. She issued a commission that every householder in London should lay out wood and make bonfires at seven in the evening to consume the corrupt airs. The sight of a Londoner's flat cap struck terror through the villages and the wells were padlocked to discourage refugees from lingering.

Thomas Dekker, a dramatist whose living ceased as the theatres were closed, describes an empty city with the rich fleeing and the physicians profiteering. Their nostrums

> had not so much a strength to hold life and soul together as a pot of Pinder's ale and a nutmeg. Their drugs turned to dirt, their simples were simple things . . . the rabble of doctors and watercasters were at their wits' end for not one of them durst peep abroad.

Churchyard and burial plots were soon filled to capacity and sextons and churchwardens made a fortune in bribes from relatives desperate to find a decent resting place for their dead. One churchwarden in Thames Street, implored for a space in his churchyard, answered mockingly that he wanted it for himself. He was buried in it within three days.

Dekker describes with horror the mass graves into which the living were sometimes thrown along with the dead:

> All ceremonial due to them was taken away, they were launched ten in one heap, twenty in another, the gallant and the beggar together, the husband saw his wife and his deadly enemy whom he hated within a pair of sheets.

The plague returned annually, usually reaching its peak in the flea month of September, until 1610. Visitors to London would delay their arrival until the first frosts of winter cleared the air. The city was half paralysed, and those who could earn a living elsewhere did so. Possibly plague was the reason for Shakespeare's removal from the Globe Theatre to Stratford.

Then once again the pestilence retreated until new generations of rats and men could be bred for the slaughter.

The conditions for plague were still present, scarcely having improved since Erasmus, a fastidious Dutchman, described English floors 'covered with rushes piled, the new on the old, for twenty years without a clearance, befouled with all manner of filth, with spillings of beer and the remains of fish, with spit and vomit, excrement and urine', a paradise for rats and fleas.

In 1625 once again the sound of clocks striking the hours was drowned by the tolling of bells for departed souls and only the coffin-makers, quacks and dog-killers prospered (dogs were thought to carry the infection in their hair – true enough in that they probably acquired the rat flea). Plague swept across London with, it was claimed, the sweet smell of a mellow apple. While the empty streets echoed to cries from the pain of the swelling buboes, the delirious ravings of the dying and the cry 'Bring out your dead', physicians profiteered, posting bills with claims for expensive cures claiming 'slight means and cheap medicines, however they promise, prove as dear as death'. Grass grew in what had been busy thoroughfares and the Dean of St Paul's decribed in graphic terms how

> the citizens fled away as out of a house on fire, and stuffed their pockets with their best ware, and threw themselves into the highways, and were not received so much as into barns, and perished so. Some of them with more money about them than would have bought the village where they died.

Fifty thousand died that year in London.

The Great Plague of London of 1665 was scarcely more severe than the plague of 1603 or 1625. At the time it was reported that the infection reached the city in a bale of silks from the Levant, shipped from Holland to a house in Long Acre, but the truth is that plague had been endemic in London for almost a century. It had been a very dry summer after severe frosts and the ground was too parched to grow more than a poor harvest as can be judged from the meadows at Acton which bore only four loads of hay that year instead of the usual forty. It is possible that the dearth of food in the countryside drove the rats into the city, packing them together until the latent infection could explode. Certainly it is true that the infection began in Highgate, Hampstead and Acton, all outlying villages on London roads. Slowly it swept eastward across the city so that it was almost over in one suburb before beginning in the next, 'like a dark cloud that passes over our heads, which as it thickens and overcasts the air at one end, clears up at the other.' It reached its worst in August and September in the crowded alleys of Southwark and the East End. 'All sorts died, but more of the good than the bad, more men than women, more of dull complexion than fair.'

The authorities argued the virtues of burning coal as opposed to wood fires in the streets to clear the air, 40 000 dogs and 200 000 cats were killed, but rats went scot-free. The people blamed the comet of the previous year, which perhaps gave rise to the legend of the plague maiden, a bright incandescence in the sky, sometimes to appear as a mortal woman to force some peasant to carry her on his shoulders as she spread the plague from village to village with immunity as his reward. With no rational explanation for the terror which haunted them, people would snatch at anything which promised a chance of protection or cure. Sapphire and amber became popular as talismans against infection, and there was a great demand for tobacco, which the boys at Eton were compelled to smoke as a defence against the pestilence.

Two-thirds of the inhabitants fled from London, famine broke out and typhus added to the victims. Although the price of bread did not rise, so few had any employment that many were prepared to take on the dangerous and hated work as watchmen of shut-up houses or searchers for the dead. Burials were supposed to be done at night but the nights became too short and coffins lay uncollected all day in the streets. In the worst week over 8000 died and before the infection had burned itself out there were 98 000 deaths, over a fifth of the population.

From time to time construction workers still dig open plague pits full of skeletons, macabre evidence of the horrors of those times, described with relish by Defoe in his *Journal of the Plague Year*. Defoe was only four years old at the time of great plague, but he capitalized on the 1720 plague of Marseilles, one of the worst in history, to scare Londoners with an account gleaned from contemporary sources. However, London was to be spared this time. The last plague in England had died out in Nottingham in 1667 (except for a few cases in Essex in 1909). All we have left are the records, the *Diaries* of Pepys and Evelyn, the legends and the folk rhymes.

| | |
|---|---|
| Ring a ring o'roses, | *(The rash.* |
| A pocket full of posies, | *Nosegays to filter the* |
| Ah-tishoo! Ah-tishoo! | *pestilential smells.* |
| We all fall down. | *Pneumonic plague kills.)* |

The dance dates from the Black Death when in France and the Netherlands men, women and children joined hands in the street and danced until they dropped to the ground from exhaustion, shrieking and calling to visions of the saints and God. Dancing manias such as St Vitus's dance, St John's dance, tarantism and the *Carmagnole* of the French Revolution seem to be a form of public expression giving release to otherwise unendurable psychological stress.

That we catch plague at all is an accident of Nature as it is a disease of rodents. And the failure of plague to return to Europe has more to do with the fate of the rat than that of the flea.

Compared with the rat, man is a recent inhabitant of the earth, but the numbers of man and rat are about equal. The black rat, *Rattus rattus,* is thought to have come to Europe with the return of the first Crusaders, and it was not long arrived before days of prayer were set aside in England for protection from its ravages. The black or sewer rat is a climber, and being smaller in size was no match for the brown rat, *Rattus norvegicus,* which did not reach Europe until 1727 when, after an earthquake, a ravenous horde swarmed across the river Volga. The brown rat was unknown to the great French naturalist Buffon in 1753 and Linnaeus did not list it in 1758, but by 1775 it had not only colonized England, it had spread to America as well. The key to this success in colonizing new territory is that rats are astonishingly prolific breeders, a female can have three to six litters a year of about ten young each time. This means that if all the offspring were able to survive, one pair of rats could produce over 350 million descendants in three years. Fortunately under normal conditions their survival rate is low, but they are able to respond quickly to any increase in territory or food supply with new generations.

Rats on their own are formidable enemies, they have even been known to cause the death of elephants by gnawing their feet and there are 3-4000 cases of rat-bites reported every year from large American cities alone. These are usually suffered by people unable to defend themselves. Infants, invalids and the unconscious can suffer gnawing of hands and feet, which occasionally results in death, but one case on record in Britain tells of a miner who visited a disused shaft in a coal-mine. He was overwhelmed by starving rats and bitten to death.

Traditionally it has been the black rat which has been the vector of plague, but the brown or Norwegian rat can also carry the bacillus. In India the brown rat was found to develop plague shortly before the black rats caught it, and it is sometimes solely responsible, as at outbreaks in Malta. The two species have distinct behaviour patterns, and the decline in incidence of the plague since the seventeenth century has been attributed in the past to the brown rat driving the black rat out of cities as is happening at present in Israel.

The black rat, *Rattus rattus,* also called the roof rat, is a much better climber than its cousin, it has a tail longer than its body, light slender hind quarters and a pointed nose. In Britain it is still common in port areas and in the sewers of big cities, and in America it thrives in the southern and Pacific coast states, but its main headquarters are now in the tropics.

The brown rat, *Rattus norvegicus,* is about a third larger in size, with a shorter tail, heavy hind quarters and a blunt muzzle, and it is a burrowing animal. In England it used to be called the Hanoverian rat as it came to London about the time of George I and it became a sport to pitch terriers against large numbers of rats in a pit. The record, according to Mayhew, was 100 rats killed in five minutes. Rat-hunting as it was called became so popular that it accounted for 100 000 rats a year in London. Rats sold for sport fetched 2s 6d to 3s a dozen before the practice was banned in 1870.

Rats were also eaten with relish on long voyages in sailing ships where fresh meat was unobtainable. They were especially popular with midshipmen in the Royal Navy where they were held to be as moist in flesh as rabbits and as well flavoured. But in general man's enmity with the rat has been complete, and he has been at great pains to exterminate it. In recent years this had been done by using a poison which is an anticoagulant (it is used as a medicine for those likely to have blood clots — but in small doses). It was developed at the Wisconsin Alumni Research Foundation and was given the name Warfarin from the initials of the foundation. Its great advantage was that rats, which are notoriously suspicious of poisons, did not connect it with their subsequent death from internal haemorrhages since the symptoms were slow to appear.

But any poison which is not 100 per cent effective carries the risk that individuals will survive and be able to breed resistant offspring which will soon dominate in the population, and in 1958 there were reports from Scotland and Shropshire which showed that resistant colonies had indeed bred. Since Warfarin was used all over Britain for rat control this was a very serious matter, and at once a *cordon sanitaire* 4·8 kilometres wide was created around the foci where all rats were vigilantly killed. In spite of these measures the resistance soon spread and in 1970 a four-year poison campaign against the 'super-rats' was finally abandoned. It is indicative of our double standards towards animals and our health that whilst Warfarin, which causes internal bleeding, has been used widely without objection, another organophosphorous poison TEPP which rats absorb from the ground through their feet, and which causes some of them to bite off their toes before dying has caused widespread human aversion and objection. In early 1974 a new poison Sorexa CR was introduced which again gave the initiative back to man, but clearly there is no likelihood of rats and the threat of plague becoming extinct.

All this may seem rather far from the subject of this book, but so far as plague is concerned rat and flea go together. In 1908 when there was a real fear of an epidemic of plague in California the Citizens' Health Committee was founded to din into the public ear that the plague is a disease of rats and transmitted to man through the medium of the flea. Just as in Camus's classic novel, *La Peste*, about an outbreak in Oran, the authorities, far from having their citizens' interests foremost in their minds, were more concerned that an admission that there was plague in San Francisco might lead to the port being declared out of-bounds to shipping and a catastrophic decline in trade. One mayor of the city refused to approve the printing of health reports and vital statistics and tried to fire four members of the Board of Health who persistently upheld the fact that plague existed in the city. All the same, after eighteen months of effort the outbreak died down chiefly because of an all-out attack on the rat population.

What was much more worrying was that not long afterwards the disease was found to be endemic amongst ground squirrels, just as it is amongst the marmots and turbagans of Central Asia. The disease in ground squirrels passes through the usual cycles of intensity from year to year, and since they live in areas which are remote from cities the danger of an infection of man is not immediate, but there have already been two small epidemics of the very dangerous and infectious pneumonic form of plague which have been traced to them. Nearly 200 species of rodents have been reported as involved in the spread of the infection. It is not a great exercise of the imagination to see how a cycle of the plague in ground squirrels could coincide with a peak in the rat population, and since there are always plenty of fleas. . . . But at least we now have the knowledge of antibiotics like strepto-mycin, chloramphenicol and sulphadiazine which can successfully be used to treat patients even with pneumonic plague, and there are now effective vaccines.

What we must guard against is the idea that plague is a thing of the past. It remains with us only waiting for the opportunity to take advantage of a weakness in hygiene to strike again. In the past it was always an accompaniment to war. Not for nothing does Macbeth at Dunsinane cry out 'Our castle's strength will laugh a siege to scorn: here let them lie, Till famine and the ague eat them up.' The fate of besieging armies was often more awful from disease than that of the besieged from hunger. A nuclear war might well provide just those conditions which plague needs.

# 8
## Lice

*We can hardly suppose that it was quartered on Adam and his
lady .... And yet as it disdained to graze the fields or lick the
dust for sustenance, where else could it have had its subsistence?*
A WRITER IN THE *Gentleman's Magazine*, 1746

Few men love a louse. Unlike the flea which has won the grudging
fascination of generations of itching victims the louse is beyond the
pale. No one describes lice as skipping merrily, no one makes a
living from their antics. To be lousy is a shameful humiliating con-
demnation. Yet the louse thrives wherever man lives, whether
Eskimo or native of the Congo, in slum and *salon*, and in Western
Europe it is on the increase. It is estimated that there are a million
and a half lousy people in Britain, and a survey in an industrial area
in 1970 revealed that 26 per cent of secondary school children had
head lice. As this edition goes to press in September 1977 there is a
national campaign to eradicate the insect. I am prepared to say now
that it will not succeed.

The head louse, just because it is unmentionable, appears to
be enjoying a social immunity aided by the fashion for unkempt
hair, the independence and ignorance of youth, and the belief
that they will not infest a clean head. As if that were not enough,
the pubic or crab louse is increasing in numbers at a rate that
has been likened to an epidemic, swept on a wave that closely
parallels the rise in cases of VD. Only the body louse is having a
hard time, forced to rely on areas of the globe where famine or
political strife ensure a continuous supply of wretchedly poor
refugees.

121

There have been times, admittedly, when lice were regarded as the pearls of poverty. Just as the Christian ascetic Simeon the stylite was said to have picked up the maggots which fell from his rotting flesh to replace them in their burrows with the exhortation to eat what God had provided for them, so did saintly men in the Middle Ages consider their bodies a haven not to be denied to the louse. After all they had heaven to look forward to as a reward for earthly sanctity, whilst the poor louse had only the pleasures of the hour. The natives of Malabar, it is said, if irritated by head lice, would call on holy men who would willingly take the lice and put them on their own heads for nourishment. In Tonga catching and eating the lice on one's parents was a sign of filial duty and affection. And Cortes watched Indians bringing gifts of small bags to Montezuma, which the avaricious Spaniard at once assumed to be full of gold dust. Instead to his astonishment and disgust he found them to be full of lice. The assumption at the time was that Indians too poor to bring any other tribute would give the harvest of their own bodies, but it is highly probable, although it spoils the story, the bags were instead full of cochineal insects which live on the Mexican cactus and yield a valuable red dye.

Tolerance of insult whether by man or parasite and mortification of the flesh to ennoble the spirit have fallen out of fashion, but the legends and the lice live on. The sheer difficulty of keeping clean in the days before looking-glasses and soap ensured the persistence of vermin.

One of the most vivid descriptions of a verminous captured army that I have read is contained in a poem by Amir Khusran Dihlant written in 1289 AD.

Their eyes were so narrow and piercing that they might have bored a hole in a brazen vessel. Their stink was more horrible than their colour. Their faces were set on their bodies as if they had no neck. Their cheeks resembled soft leathern bottles, full of wrinkles and knots. Their noses extended from cheek-bone to cheek-bone. Their nostrils resembled rotten graves, and from them the hair descended as far as the lips.

Their moustaches were of extravagant length. They had but scanty beards about their chins. Their chests, of a colour half black, half white, were so covered with lice that they looked like sesame growing on a bad soil. Their whole body, indeed, was covered with these insects, and their skin was as rough-grained as chagreen leather, fit only to be converted into shoes.

These were the 'Tartar infidels' — Mongols who had captured the writer four years previously and he had little cause to like them. It is interesting that he notes that they shaved their heads.

Herodotus tells us that Egyptian priests shaved their heads every three days to remain uncontaminated, while those with less time for such rigorous toilet actually began to approve of their parasites. In primitive Mediterranean communities it is still considered a sign of virility to be lousy, and it seems that this was a common belief in the Middle Ages. Even Linnaeus believed lice protected children from disease. One traveller to northern Siberia recorded how the young women flirtatiously threw their lice at him, anxious to demonstrate their love with tokens of their serious intentions.

It was in Hurdenburg in Sweden where the louse reached his apotheosis. Each year when the mayor was to be elected the eligible notables of the town would sit at a round table touching it with their beards. A louse was then dropped in the centre, and the man whose beard it climbed was forthwith declared mayor for the coming year.

In England, by the seventeenth century, the public attitude had crystallized to disgust. Thomas Mouffet, father of the arachnidaphobic Miss Muffet of the nursery rhyme, collected a work called *Theatrum Insectorum*, a sort of encyclopedia of the knowledge of insects of the time published in 1634. He is not enthusiastic about the louse:

> It is a beastly creature and known better in Innes and armies than it is welcome . . . . If you rub them gently between your fingers, you shall see them foursquare and somewhat harder than fleas, whence in the dark you may easily find the

difference .... As for dressing the body: all Ireland is noted
for this, that it swarms almost with lice. But that this proceeds
from the beastliness of the people and want of cleanly women
to wash them, is manifest, because the English that are more
careful to dress themselves, changing and washing their shirts
often, have escaped the plague. Hence it is that armies and
prisons are so full of lice, the sweat being corrupted by
wearing always the same clothes, and from this arises matter
for their origin, by the mediation of heat.

Despite the misguided report of their spontaneous generation
there is certainly some truth in this description related to body
lice. Since they lay their eggs in clothes, and the eggs are killed
by both cold and heat, washing and ironing one's linen is the
best cure, and it is this practice which has almost extinguished
the body louse in Britain, while the head louse which cements its
egg to the hair continues to thrive.

Believing that lice derived from sweat put Mouffet to some
trouble to explain away nits (eggs of the head louse) which he
treats in a different chapter as 'insects without feet'. 'The
philosopher affirms they proceed from the copulation of lice and
are therefore called their eggs ... as the jasmine brings forth
flowers without seed, so lice bring forth eggs without young ones
in them.' It was left for later religious philosophers to speculate
on the difficult problem that if God made lice, which feed only
on human blood, at the creation they would have detracted
somewhat from the pleasures of the Garden of Eden.

Since Mouffet our quest for knowledge of the louse has been
spurred on by the realization that it is one of man's deadliest
enemies. Just as the flea spreads plague so does the louse spread
typhus, and it is no exaggeration to say that typhus, like plague,
has changed the history of the world. As an uncomfortably
recent example, at the time of World War I typhus killed three
million people in eastern Europe, particularly in Russia and
Poland. Russian soldiers were said to de-louse their garments by
putting them on ants' nests.

Almost all our knowledge of the behaviour of the insects has been gleaned from the sordid and heroic procedure of allowing them to feed on the experimenter's body, confined in pill-boxes against the skin. And several experimenters on typhus have paid for their knowledge with their lives.

Lice are classified in the order *Phthiraptera,* subdivided as the biting lice Mallophaga (literally wool-eaters), which feed on feathers and the debris of skin and hair, and the sucking lice, Anoplura (unarmed tail or stingless), which suck blood from the capillaries of the host. The Mallophaga are widespread parasites of birds and mammals although they do not colonize man and it is likely that the blood-sucking louse developed from them, sacrificing a degree of independence for the constant availability of hot meals.

Of the seven families of Anoplura only one parasitizes Primates — man and monkeys — called the Pediculidae (little lice). They are wingless, and flat from front to back perhaps as a result of their ancestors' need to live amongst feathers; they have claws adapted to clinging to hair and retractable mouth-parts to pierce the skin and suck blood. They are, except for the camel louse, the only family of lice that have retained eyes and consequently they behave differently in light and dark. Human lice are exclusive to man, but they will happily feed on pigs for a few days just as the flea and chigoe will, but there is probably no natural transfer between man and animals. However the spider monkeys of the South American jungles and east India have a species of *Pediculus* that is very similar to ours, which must have been transferred in man's remote past because the common ancestors of the monkey and ourselves are too far removed for similar lice to have evolved. The natural course of evolution is for related hosts to evolve related parasites, for example the ground squirrels of North America are related to but distinct from those which live in Siberia while their lice appear to be identical.

Lice themselves have no insect parasites but their bodies do harbour micro-organisms. All sucking lice have strange organs called *mycetonae,* stomach discs containing symbiotic organisms which remain throughout the life of the larva and male

The Life That Lives on Man

louse. In the female they enter the eggs via the wall of the oviduct and so reach the next generation, and it is thought that they supply vitamins which are deficient in the blood of the host. These strange organisms, bacteria and perhaps yeasts, have been studied very little, but certainly neither adult nor egg can survive without them.

There are two genera of lice found on man and only one species of each, although there are over 200 other species of sucking lice. *Pediculus humanus* and *Phthirus pubis* are closely related but are adapted to different modes of life and different areas of the human habitat. Adults of both kinds have five-jointed antennae, pigmented eyes, and are obligate parasites living exclusively on blood. They are only able to survive in close contact with their host and are well adapted to evade his attentions. The force needed to pop a louse is about 500 000 times its own weight.

*Pediculus humanus* is the species which includes both the head louse, *P.h. capitis,* and the body louse, *P.h. humanus.* The two varieties are so similar in appearance that it is very hard to tell specimens apart without being able to study their habits. In general the body louse is about 20 per cent larger than the head louse, the largest female body louse being about 4 millimetres long and the smallest male head louse 2 millimetres, with a full range between. These are, of course, immense compared with mites, and are easily visible to the naked eye, so they have become adept at concealing themselves either in the hair or in the seams of underclothing. The two varieties can be interbred experimentally but their behaviour and indeed their success as parasites are very different, and it seems likely that the body louse is an adaptation of the older head louse which has taken place since man began to wear clothes. The head louse, which spends all its life in close proximity to the skin, cementing its eggs to hair near the scalp, diverged in its habits and began instead to lay eggs cemented to the fibres of clothing. Primitive tribes who wear no clothing have no body lice, although in some cases lice are found to live and lay their eggs on the only available extra cover — strings of beads or other ornaments on necklaces.

There is no doubt that head lice have been with us for a long time; they have been found on American Indian mummies several thousand years old. It has even been suggested that the presence of lice in the Americas similar to those found on the Chinese and the Eskimos of the Aleutian Islands is a further support to the theory that man reached the Americas by crossing the Bering Straits. Charles Darwin reported that lice that decided to move from Hawaiians to English sailors died before the week was out, but it is now generally accepted that the louse will modify its colour early in life according to the pigment of its host's skin.

There is no doubt that there are different races of head lice which have evolved on the different races of man. For example the European variety is at a great disadvantage when it finds itself in the flat cross-section hair of a Negro which its claws cannot grip properly. This is why head lice are comparatively rare at present on children of Negro descent in Britain. The African head louse by contrast has a claw shape adapted to the flat negroid hair. The American variety, which by now has been extensively interbred with the European, has special modifications to its breathing apparatus, and the Chinese head louse is also structurally distinct. Despite these differences all the races of lice can interbreed.

In terms of survival rate of offspring, resistance to change in temperature and survival without food, the body louse is much more successful than the head louse. But the head louse is by far the most common in industrial societies and so I will describe it first.

Lice are hemimetabolic insects, which means that they do not go through a complete metamorphosis, they have no pupal form unlike the flea. Fortunately for us the egg or nit of the head louse is surprisingly large, nearly a millimetre long. It is invariably cemented to the hair near the scalp and is a yellow-whitish colour through which the embryo can be seen. Strangely most nits are found on girls in the area just over or behind the ears, but on boys near the top of the head. They hatch after eight to nine days, and since hair grows at the rate of third of a millimetre a day the egg is already clear of the scalp before it hatches. The outer end of the egg has a circular flat lid pierced with cavities to allow air to reach the embryo. When the young louse has developed it pierces the lid of the egg with its proboscis, since it has no teeth to bite its way out. It then swallows air which it ejects beneath it, ingeniously forcing itself out of the eggshell by compressed air. The cement is so secure that the empty 'nits' usually remain attached to the hair until the hair is shed and there is no known solvent which will remove them. So the nits which are frequently seen dangling on long hairs are almost always empty, and look opalescent, translucent and flat.

The nymph which emerges needs a blood meal at once. The blood it sucks is visible through the cuticle so that the feeding insects have been likened to tiny rubies; though few have admired them as beautiful. There are always three moults and the three types of nymph appear very similar except in length. Each requires a blood meal before further development can begin, otherwise it dies within a day or two. Within eight or nine days from hatching the adult emerges, a greyish insect which has adapted during the nymphal stages to the colour of the hair in which it lives so that the lice of blondes are paler than those of brunettes.

The abdomen of the louse is divided into seven distinct segments and the three pairs of legs are modified for grasping hair. A strong curved claw clamps the hair against a thumb-like projection further up the leg, and anyone who has tried to remove a louse will know how strong the grip is. Each antenna has three different types of sense organ; pegs, tufts and tactile hairs, each specialized to a different function. As a louse moves it waves its antennae from side to side with a characteristic movement. The male is generally smaller than the female and it has larger front legs with a stouter claw and thumb which it uses to grasp the hind leg of the female during copulation.

Between the last moult and egg laying only one or two days elapse and the female will then lay fertile eggs for up to twenty-eight days at the rate of eight or ten eggs every night, cementing them to hairs with a secretion from glands either side of the oviduct. Although the lifespan of the adult is as long as four weeks in experimental conditions, it is likely that ten days is a more realistic average in the wild where the human host is the only predator.

The mouth-parts of a louse are normally withdrawn into a pouch in the head and are not visible, but when feeding a small tube is extended with teeth which rotate outwards to grip the skin of the sufferer. Then three lance-like stylets are jabbed in and out by muscles to pierce the skin and tissues of the dermis. The capillary blood pressure is then high enough to squirt blood into the mouth of the insect through the stylets; it is then pumped into the gut where it soon turns a dark purplish colour clearly visible through the cuticle. The bite is painless but the saliva of the insect, which probably acts as an anti-coagulant and is injected via the stylets, causes irritation within eight or ten hours.

If an individual has not been bitten previously each bite produces a tiny red spot that does not itch until after the first week, giving the louse not only time to get clear but ample time to lay eggs. In the second or third week of an infestation, as with other insect bites, symptoms of sensitization begin to appear whose severity depends greatly on the individual concerned. Some will suffer from severe swelling while others may only have small red spots and hardly any itching. Lice need to feed regularly, about every three hours, and will die if starved for two days.

The degree of infestation that some individuals will tolerate is remarkable. In the nineteenth century in Poland the custom of wearing tight fur caps and the superstitious belief that a lousy scalp was healthy lead to the common occurrence of *Plica polonica,* a filthy inflamed stinking scalp with the hair matted into a sticky moist mass in which lice thrived.

'Clean' parents react with such disgust and distress at finding their children infested that it suggests that the condition is rare and shameful. But in practice a child can catch lice as easily as it can catch measles. In some posh private girls' schools in

England the pupils' heads are searched every time they have been on public transport. It is referred to as the elephant hunt. One outbreak in a boys' school was traced to the felt pads of the earphones in the language laboratory.

Lice have always been more common in comunities living in close proximity and the difference between towns and country is striking. The first time the lousiness of the urban population impinged on the middle-class consciousness in England was at the start of World War II. As a precaution against the likelihood that there would be intensive bombing of London and other major cities by the Nazis, plans were made under the Civil Defence Act of 1939 for voluntary evacuation of children and mothers with babies. They were compulsorily billeted on families in the country.

Up to that time a steady improvement in social legislation and wages had fostered a sense of complacency in Britain about the state of the slums. The first main exodus occurred in September 1939 at the end of the summer holidays when 735 000 unaccompanied schoolchildren and 260 000 young children accompanied by the mothers flooded into the countryside.

A howl of outrage arose at once. According to a letter in *The Times* a fortnight later 'Complaints are pouring in about half-savage, verminous, and wholly illiterate children from some slums who have been billeted on clean homes. Stories with which one cannot but sympathize are told of mattresses and carpets polluted, of wilful despoliation and dirt that one would associate only with untrained animals.' The reluctance with which these children were welcomed into homes is vividly described by Evelyn Waugh in his novel *Put Out More Flags*.

The greatest complaints were against the mothers of young children. An official study by the Women's Group on Public Welfare (published by OUP, 1943) reported:

It was said that they were dirty, verminous, idle and extravagant; that they could not hold a needle and did not know the rudiments of cooking and housecraft, and that they had no control over their young children, who were untrained and animal in their habits. Some of these women were said to be foul-mouthed, bullying, and abusive, given to drinking and frequenting public houses, insanitary in their habits and loose in their morals. In almost every reception area there were householders who said, after a first experience, that they would defy the law rather than take such persons into their homes again.

The press concluded that the problem of teaching the principles of decent living to the future mothers of the race remained to be solved.

The evacuees themselves did not appreciate this fastidious reception and after three months 88 per cent of the mothers had returned home to brave the bombs, which of course at that stage of the war had not begun to fall.

Kenneth Mellanby, then a medical entomologist, describes in his book, *Human Guinea Pigs,* how he came to do research on infestation figures. He had

assumed that 'blimpish' country dwellers in a hitherto protected environment had greatly exaggerated a very unimportant problem which had been thrust upon their notice. When, however, I came to examine children recently taken into hospital I soon came to the conclusion that any misrepresentation on the part of the newspapers at the time of evacuation had been to minimize the problem. I was appalled at the number of children with lousy heads.

Mellanby found from a survey of 60 000 individuals that the heaviest infestation in boys was in the pre-school years. Forty-two per cent had lice in industrial cities but only 8 per cent in the country, and amongst city-living girls half of them were infested from one year old till the age of thirteen. The longer-lasting infestation of girls was blamed on the current fashion for permanent waves, also given to children, who were then discouraged from combing their hair. The figures were three times as high as those from the school Medical Officers' reports and the very high numbers of pre-school children infested meant

that campaigns carried out at school alone would have little
result. Two out of three girls of school age in Liverpool were
lousy, and Mellanby also found that the larger the families, the
more likely they were to be verminous.

This disgustingly high incidence compares with figures from
Mexican villages studied in 1944 which revealed 79-91 per cent
lousy.

During the war vigorous efforts were made in Britain to
eradicate the louse population and they were partly successful.
The percentage of all girls infested fell from 40 in 1940 to 11 in
1963. But in 1970 Dr R. J. Donaldson, the Medical Officer of
Health for Teesside, decided to take a closer look at disturbing
reports from schools in his area. He commissioned a survey
which showed that the reported rate of 5·7 per cent in 1969 was
ridiculously low compared with the actual situation. In fact 30
per cent of children in some primary schools were infested and
26 per cent of secondary school children in two schools. Overall
the infestation rate was 16 per cent which meant that one child
in seven had lice or nits — any one class might be expected to
have up to six children lousy.

Following a campaign on local television and in the press,
eighteen extra staff were taken on to help the school nurses
recognize and treat the problem. Within a year and a half the
infestation rate in primary schools had been cut to 3 per cent,
but not before it had been discovered that the lice were resistant
to the traditional methods of treatment with gamma benzine
hexachloride insecticides. Alternative methods recommended by
parents varied from shaving their children's heads to fly sprays
and the use of 'anti-mate' sold to keep bitches free from
unwanted litters. But it was clear that the major cause of the
epidemic was the parents' ignorance that the problem still
existed. Both publicity and the use of a malathion-based
insecticide which had been developed by the London School of
Hygiene were needed before the infestation was effectively
curbed.

An adult louse travels easily from one head of hair to another
simply by walking across touching hair when children play

games or huddle together. But it is still disputed whether they are also transferred on hats, combs, the backs of chairs and other inanimate objects. On Teesside having removed the schools as a source of infection it became apparent that it was a family problem. The belief that some children 'breed' lice dies hard, and too often it is the parents themselves who harbour the residual population which reinfests the children. But scarcely a single father on Teesside would allow himself to be inspected. The normal head louse population is less than ten insects, and it appears that light infestations are often not recognized. Over 1000 lice were twice found on unfortunate children in the East End of London in 1941, but the record for head lice was found on a woman evacuee in Burma who had 1434 lice. She had been insect-free only three months before. I have seen a photograph of a mummified Indian found in the desert of Peru that had hair so festooned with nits that each hair looked like a necklace.

An infestation usually begins with the transfer of an adult louse and there is a high mortality rate in the larval forms. The notion that it is sufficient to wash hair to keep it free from lice is entirely unfounded. If immersed in water a louse seals off its breathing holes down each side of its body and survives unharmed.

In 1974 Birmingham admitted to an infestation rate of 7 per cent of school children, but going on Mellanby's principle that half remain undiscovered and a further half inhabit pre-school children it is likely that altogether there are a million and a half people in Britain with lousy heads. There is no reason to believe that large cities elsewhere in the world should be any cleaner than those in Britain, indeed with free medical care it is likely that the British are better off.

But in general the British attitude is to prefer to pretend that the problem does not exist. Dr Donaldson told me that after he had discussed his Teesside campaign on my television programme he was severely criticized by other Medical Officers of Health for unnecessarily alarming the public.

Most of the information on the behaviour of lice has been found from studying body lice. The fact that they lay their eggs for preference attached to garments, usually along the seams next to the skin, means that they are subjected to a wider range of temperature than those of head lice. It also makes them more vulnerable. The incubation period of these eggs varies from six days at body temperature to nineteen days at 24°C. Taking clothes off at night does not cause a sufficient temperature change to kill them but washing clothes in hot water and particularly ironing the seams will destroy both eggs and lice.

The female body louse lays up to 250 eggs and allowing for some mortality of eggs and larvae it has been calculated that a single fertilized female can result in a colony of 15 000 viable females, of which 10 000 are eggs, in eighty days. The highest count ever found was 3800 body lice on one person.

A number of unsavoury experiments have been carried out on volunteers to see how lice behave. As a result we know that they like the dark and prefer the smell of man and their fellows, and it is likely that they colonize new individuals during the night, attracted by bodily warmth. If released next to the skin under a woollen vest they travel about 30 centimetres in two hours, but can cover over 30 centimetres a minute on the flat, presumably hurrying to reach shelter. One experimenter who introduced lice into occupied sleeping bags found that they were more likely to feel at home if the victim was wearing woollen rather than poplin pyjamas. But a third of his lice escaped to make forays into the unknown.

Since body lice lay their eggs along the seams of clothing it is easy to see why heavy infestations are associated with armies and refugees and prisons where people cannot change their clothes and live huddled in close proximity. In one London hostel where a third of the inmates had lice, a third of their beds also were found to contain lice although the sheets were regularly changed. If the beds were left empty for a night they were far less likely to be infested.

In the ordinary way lice are protected from variations in temperature by their close contact with the human skin, and in return for an abundant food supply they have forfeited the ability to survive independently. Without their human host they quickly starve or die from cold. It is often remarked that in Mediterranean countries and India there are less lice in hot weather — they cannot resist dry heat.

There is a Turkish expression often used in heroic ballads which claims, as an expression of stark terror, that a man's lice ran to his feet. It is in fact true that if a man has a fever or sweats severely adult lice will move rapidly away in search of another host. If a louse is put on blotting paper and moves to a damp patch it stops with its antennae alone overlapping the damp area and at once turns back. It may be that the tuft organs on the antennae are sensitive to moisture. But it is not just a question of lice not liking to get their feet wet, it is an instinctive protection mechanism developed to aid their survival. A blood meal from a host perspiring with fever might contain micro-organisms fatal to the louse. So far as man is concerned this flight from a fever-stricken host is of the greatest importance in the spread of the disease typhus.

## Typhus

Typhus is caused by an organism called *Rickettsia prowazeki* after an American and an Austrian who both contracted the disease while they were studying it. Both men died from its effects. (Ricketts, as I mentioned in Chapter 5, had already showed that the deadly Rocky Mountain spotted fever was caused by a tick.) Classical typhus is passed to man by the louse, a fact established by Charles Nicolle in 1909 in a famous series of experiments when he showed first that typhus could be transferred from a man to a chimpanzee by injecting it with the man's blood, and then that the infection could be transmitted by feeding fresh lice on an infected monkey and then on uninfected monkeys. It was not realized until later that the disease is very seldom passed to man by the bite of the louse, unlike plague which is inoculated by the bite of the flea.

The reason for this is that the Rickettsiae multiply in the gut of the louse which swells and bursts allowing huge numbers of the organism to appear in the excrement of the insect which dries to a fine black powder. The louse dies within twelve days of infection, but if the faeces are kept dry and at room temperature the organism can remain virulent for as long as sixty-six days. It infects man by getting into his bloodstream through scratches often caused by the irritation of the louse-bites, or through the lungs, the conjunctiva of the eye, or the mucous membrane (especially in localities like the Andes where lice are habitually killed by biting).

Rickettsiae are bacillus-like elliptical organisms which come mid-way in characteristics between virus and bacterum, they can live both inside and outside the cells of the host, are clearly seen under a microscope, and are frequently found in the bodies of many kinds of insect. Typhus is caused by an intra-cellular variety, and they differ from ordinary bacteria in their response to staining techniques and in that they will only multiply within cells both in tissue-culture and in the living animal. They will not grow on dead media like the agar plates used to culture bacteria.

Typhus can only spread to epidemic proportions in a population mostly infested with body lice. In the laboratory the head louse will also pass on the disease and although so far there is no evidence to implicate it in natural outbreaks, it remains an ominous threat. While the human mortality rate from typhus is from 30 to 60 per cent, it is invariably fatal to the louse itself and this raises a series of interesting questions. Once again, these involve the principle of parasitism that the longer a parasitic association has continued the less harm it is likely to do the host.

Clearly it is not in the interests of the parasite to kill off its food supply. So the fact that man tolerates the Rickettsia of typhus better than the louse implies that the louse has only relatively recently been associated with the disease. There are other puzzles. Although lice are distributed world-wide, typhus is a disease of temperate climates which does not occur in India and the tropics. And why has the disease declined since 1870? Why was there no outbreak on the Western Front in World War I when soldiers were lousy and louse-borne trench fever was widespread? In 1917 the Second Army had 10 000 casualties admitted for inflammation of the skin, most of them caused by secondary infection of louse-bites, but typhus did not occur. Yet between 1917 and 1923 there were three million deaths from typhus in European Russia.

Since the typhus organism is so lethal to the louse there has been considerable speculation about the origin of epidemics. Where was the reservoir from which the disease could develop? Then in the 1920s it was discovered that there were two types of typhus, one from Mexico and America and the other from south-east Europe. The former came to be identified as murine typhus as it was also traced in mice and rats. It is now thought likely that the Rickettsiae were originally confined to rodents and were passed between them by the rat flea and the rat louse *Polyplax spinulosus*. The organism causes no harm to the rat flea *X. cheopis* and although it will survive for long periods in the brain of rats it causes no serious sickness. From the evolutionary point of view this seems to be the older disease and it is also likely that classical epidemic typhus derived from it. There are isolated human cases of murine typhus where the infection can be traced back to rats and it has a much milder course than classical typhus. It is perhaps only because classical typhus is so fatal to the human louse and because the gut of the louse is such a fertile medium in which the organism can multiply that it has become so important an influence in man's history. Nevertheless, once the first infected rat flea carried the disease to man it is likely that man himself has been the true reservoir providing the habitat which gives refuge to the Rickettsiae between outbreaks. This conclusion was supported by an investigation of immigrants to the USA from central Europe.

Thirty per cent of these immigrants, who had entered the USA twenty-five years before, had antibodies in their blood specific for *R. prowazeki* whereas their children did not. It was then found that the organism could be isolated from the lymphnodes of healthy immigrants who had lived for a generation in America, and it became clear sub-clinical infections could remain hidden in the population for very long periods. A lapse of immunity owing to another type of infection, or a variety of possible causes, could result in the organisms multiplying in the bloodstream. Then it only requires one louse to begin cross-infection.

The symptoms of typhus at first resemble, and are often mistaken for, those of influenza. The temperature rises quickly to about 39.5°C with a severe headache, chills, pains in the limbs and depression; the rash only appears on the fourth or fifth day on the shoulders and trunk — as pink spots which later become a deep brownish-red, spreading outwards to the hands and feet but rarely to the face; delirium and extreme weakness follow. Susceptibility to the disease varies with age. A severe outbreak will be uniformly fatal to those over sixty but only 50 per cent of fifty-year-olds will succumb, and the mortality drops rapidly to 5 per cent for those under twenty. In America the recurrence of childhood typhus amongst immigrants from eastern Europe was called Brill's disease. It was first described among the Jews of New York in 1898 and was not identified until 1906 by an immigrant doctor from Poland.

Although reputed to be responsible for the plague of Athens in 430–428 BC, the first historical epidemic of typhus which can be identified with reasonable certainty appears to have been in a monastery near Salerno, but reliable records do not begin until the fifteenth century, owing to the difficulty of identifying the symptoms of diseases which frequently struck together at populations already weakened by chronic ill health and malnutrition. It appears that in 1489 a contingent of soldiers carried the disease with them from Cyprus to Spain where the forces of Don Fernando were besieging the Moors at Granada. By the beginning of 1490, 20 000 soldiers had died from the disease, compared with only 3 000 from enemy action. A second epidemic which swept Spain from 1557 to 1570 was blamed on the Moors who had been defeated and were being dispersed by royal decree, and it depopulated the greater part of the Iberian peninsula.

Fifty years earlier the disease had played a decisive part in the defeat of the French Army besieging Naples. Within thirty days an army of 25 000 was reduced to 4000, a retreat began which was quickly turned to rout, and in 1530 Charles V was crowned ruler of the Roman empire. It is significant that both of these outbreaks were connected with armies camped for a long siege where conditions would have been extremely squalid.

For over a century as the armies of the Italians, Spanish, French, Germans, Swedish, Hungarians and Turks fought to and fro across Europe typhus was the only real victor, and it soon followed the Spanish to the New World. In Britain it first appeared as *Morbus carcerorum* or gaol fever, which soon took a dread hold on the imagination of the public through the outbreaks at 'Black Assizes'.

The first of the minor epidemics that were a direct result of the appalling conditions in which prisoners were kept and the length they had to await trial occurred at Cambridge in 1522 and was blamed on 'the savour of the prisoners or the filth of the house'. In 1577 a second outbreak occurred at Oxford which is described in the register of Merton College. A Catholic bookbinder, Rowland Jencks, was thrown into prison for being too outspoken in criticism of the government, profaning the word of God and abusing his ministers, and staying away from church. Two or three of the inmates of the prison had died in their chains a few days before the trial at which Jencks was condemned to have his ears cut off. In court the infection spread and within a few weeks almost all the members of the jury were dead as well as the Lord Chief Baron, the Sheriff and the Undersheriff. A hundred scholars of the university died and 'not a few' townsmen — about 500. The outbreak was blamed on the smell of the gaol 'where the prisoners had been long close and nastily kept' and Sir Francis Bacon came to the conclusion that the stinks must 'have some similitude with man's body and so insinuate themselves'. An observation not so far from the truth considering that no one at that time had the slightest information on airborne contagion by micro-organisms. Less fair-minded individuals blamed the Catholics of Louvain for compounding diabolic and papistical airs which were smuggled into the city. Jencks, though deprived of his ears, escaped with his life and lived for another thirty-three years as a baker in France.

The Chamberlain of the city of Exeter recounts another story of an epidemic whose precise origin can be deduced. In 1586 Sir Bernard Drake had captured a Portuguese fishing boat returning from the Newfoundland Banks and he brought his prize into Dartmouth. Thirty-eight wretched fishermen who had committed no other crime than to belong to a nation with which England was at war were sent 'unto the castell of Exon, and there were cast into the deepe pit and stinking dungeon'. They were soon infected and some died while a serious illness spread to the other inmates killing many. At the time of the assizes shortly afterwards

> Manie of them were so weak and sicke that they were not able to goe nor stand; but were carried from the gaole to the place of judgement, some upon hand barrowes ... none pitied them more than the lords justices themselves, and especially the lord chief justice himself; who ordered better care of prisoners and more frequent trials.
>
> And howsoever the matter fell out, and by what occasion it happened, an infection followed upon manie and a great number of such as were there in the court, and especially upon such as were nearest to them.

After an incubation period of fourteen days the disease attacked not only the prisoners, but killed the judge, three knights including the hapless Sir Bernard Drake, and eleven of the twelve jury. 'Of the plebeian and common people died verie manie, and especially constables, reeves, and tithing men.' Typhus raged throughout Devon for six months.

From these accounts one must come to the conclusion that in the sixteenth century not only common people but also the scholars of Oxford were lousy. Isaac Newton a century later in his tortured *Confessions* lists the sins he believes he has committed while studying at Cambridge and includes 'lying about a louse: Deceiving my chamberfellow of the knowledge of him that took him for a sot.'

Typhus also had a profound influence on the outcome of the Civil War. In 1643 King Charles I paused at Oxford, delaying a march on London. The Parliamentary Army led by Essex was ordered to attack, but both armies, each of 20 000 men, were routed by typhus without ever engaging each other. The King was forced to abandon his plan of advancing on London, and Essex occupied Reading.

Typhus was considered to be an inseparable accompaniment to war but gaol fever was blamed on bad air, and the remedy proposed by the Reverend Stephen Hales, a Twickenham parson, was to install windmills to increase ventilation. In 1752 he had one erected on Newgate gaol (which had been rebuilt originally by Dick Whittington in the fifteenth century). Two years before there had been a severe outbreak of typhus following a trial at the Old Bailey next door. It was rumoured that two men fell dead in Newgate when the first blast of fresh air struck them. Hales had already been made a Fellow of the Royal Society for his investigations into blood pressure which he measured for the first time in the leg of a horse, and he went on to fit ventilators on slave ships, which to some extent reduced the terrible mortality on the voyage across the Atlantic.

Lice and typhus had become a very serious problem on ships. In the Royal Navy it was not uncommon for a third of the ship's company to die after a call in port from 'ship-fever'. One of the opponents of the idea that ventilation cured typhus was James Lind, a physician to the Royal Naval Hospital at Haslar. He was convinced that the infection was carried both on the bodies of seamen and by their clothes and other kinds of fabrics and he recognized that outbreaks could spread from ships through the hospitals to the surrounding population. He drew attention to one outbreak which killed seventeen out of twenty-three people who had been refitting tents used for typhus patients, and recommended fumigation with smoke as a preventive measure. More important he ordered thorough cleaning and the airing of all clothes and bedding on deck. This, and his insistence that nurses and physicians should change their clothes before leaving the hospital, must have saved many lives in spite of his ignorance of the rôle of the louse.

The disease had been endemic in Ireland certainly since the beginning of the eighteenth century and pockets of infection remain there to this day, but during the great Irish epidemic of 1816–19 there were 700 000 cases recorded among six million inhabitants. Both in England and Ireland the outbreaks are notably connected with war or famine drawing the population out of their homes into huddles of refugees where the vector insects breed. Similarly an outbreak in London in 1862 came partly as the result of an economic depression which put many out of work and their homes.

But from 1870 the disease began to retreat; every five years the incidence of cases fell by half in a geometrical progression so that 4000 deaths annually in England and Wales in 1870 had become only two in 1918. It can only be assumed that the louse population suffered a catastrophic decline in the same period. Possibly this was the result of piped water and the availability of cheap machine-woven clothes so that changing clothes became common practice for the first time.

Typhus never reached the Western Front probably because in 1910 it was realized that it was a louse-borne disease, so that the Central Powers took great care not to move troops there from the east where the first outbreaks began as early as November 1914 in Serbia. There an epidemic was at its height by April and killed 150 000 people including 30 000 Austrian prisoners, yet the Austrians did not attack the disabled country, so greatly did the generals fear the disease. They could not have forgotten that of the twenty-five million men said to have died as the result of Napoleon's campaigns many more were killed by typhus than by engagement with the enemy. Only in Russia, disrupted by political revolution as well as war, did the disease become a plague.

The lesson of five million deaths from typhus during and after World War I was not lost on the German generals. Research into a typhus (*Fleckfieber*) vaccine was authorized to be carried out in concentration camps. The results were published openly in 1943 in the journal *Zeitschrift für Hygiene und Infektionskrankheiten*. They were carried out by Dr E. Dring who used prisoners in exactly the same fashion as other laboratory workers would use rats. He prepared different kinds of anti-sera and then deliberately infected prisoners with Rickettsiae. Some of them had been given anti-sera of different kinds and others had not, so that their responses to the infection could be compared. Those who recovered were said to have been released or given favoured treatment, but about 250 prisoners died; including most of those who had been the unprotected 'controls'. The fact that the results were published meant that they became the basis for both German and Allied anti-typhus vaccine policy. The Germans did not have DDT (which made the Allies' need for a vaccine far less important) and it could be argued that the 250 lives sacrificed might have saved hundreds of thousands of others. But Dr Dring did not wait to have judgement passed on him and the ethics of his experiments. He committed suicide before he could be brought to trial by the Allies.

Kenneth Mellanby made a study of concentration camp experiments after the war, and the information here comes from his account. This was probably the only item of Nazi concentration camp medical research that had a possible lasting benefit for mankind.

DDT or, more accurately, $(C_6H_4Cl)_2CHCCl_3$ was discovered to be a powerful insecticide by the Geigy Company in Switzerland in 1942, and it was carefully examined for toxicity, by the standards of the time, before being issued to the Allied forces where it was used in massive amounts. Up to one ounce of 10 per cent dust was recommended to be used in winter clothing and impregnated washproof underclothes were used on a large scale by the British forces. It completely transformed the threat of typhus to troops.

It was ready at hand to combat the last large European outbreak that began in Naples in 1943 when the disease again took advantage of wartime disruption to add another 2000 deaths to its victims. Tens of thousands of Neapolitans responded to intense propaganda from press and pulpit and reported to dusting stations where DDT was pumped into their clothing.

At the same time the risk of the outbreak spreading to Britain was taken very seriously by the health authorities and special anti-typhus squads were formed and trained to de-louse port areas. But they were not needed as DDT alone proved to be enough. Without DDT it is unlikely that the Naples outbreak could have been controlled, and the city would have been depopulated.

Avicenna recommended mercury ointment against crab lice nine centuries ago — it's ineffective — and favourite remedies have varied from butter smeared on the seams of clothing by the Carpathians, to a tramp who used axle grease and blue vitriol. But DDT was the first weapon which really worked. Now the same medical entomologists who held it to be the answer to their dreams see its effect slowly eroded as one species after another becomes resistant to it. The body louse and the head louse are now resistant to both organochlorine insecticides, DDT and gamma BHC, and will happily breed in the powder. The fact that head lice can also carry typhus and are now inhabiting such a huge percentage of the population should be disquieting to all of us, although the disease can now be treated successfully with chloramphenicol or aureomycin.

Until recently, the two presently effective agents against lice, carbaryl and malathion (on no account use the garden variety as it is impure and toxic), carbamate and organo-phosphorous agents which have the added advantage that they kill louse eggs as well as adults, were being squandered by piece-meal use by local authorities doing at best a holding operation, giving just the right conditions for the lice to acquire immunity. There is probably less than ten years before resistance develops to these chemicals in which to mount an all-out attack on the louse population to reduce it to an insignificant level.

Now, however, a country-wide campaign is being launched as children return to school. But the lesson from the war years was that an eradication campaign cannot be carried out solely in schools because of the reservoir of lice on under-fives and parents. It may well be that public education will prove to be the best insecticide. If so it is high time it started.

A heavy infestation of body lice can lead to a thickening and darkening of the skin known as 'vagabonds' disease' and extreme infestations by head lice can result in the hair becoming matted with debris from the scalp forming crusts under which lice multiply to an extraordinary extent. Both these conditions are still found in Britain.

Lice can also carry other diseases such as plague, and the Andean Indians get a plague infection of the tonsils as another result of their habit of crushing lice between their teeth.

Louse-borne trench fever is caused by an extracellular, rod-shaped organism *Rickettsia quintana* which is harmless to the louse, in contrast to the agent for typhus. It usually appears clinically as at least two attacks of acute fever and was extremely prevalent in World War I, affecting not only the troops but all those who came into contact with the louse or its faeces, for example by handling blankets. After a man has had trench fever he can infect lice for months, but the disease has since died out completely, although there were several outbreaks on the Eastern Front in World War II amongst the German Army.

Relapsing fever is another louse-borne disease caused by the spirochaete *Borrelia recurrentis,* a spiral-shaped organism capable of rapid movement. If a louse drinks blood from an infected man, six days later the spirochaete appears in the blood of the insect which circulates freely in the body cavity bathing the internal organs. The louse appears to suffer no harm and it will not transfer the spirochaete by its bite. But if the louse is crushed — as is frequently done between the fingernails — the organism is then released to be scratched into the skin. It causes high temperatures, relapses are common, and mortality can be as high as 30 per cent. It was formerly a cause of serious epidemics, but it can now be treated with chloramphenicol. There were hundreds of thousands of cases in the Balkan states in 1920, but the incidence had dropped to zero by 1925. During World War II there was a further epidemic in French North Africa, Egypt, the Sudan, Kenya and Asia. For the success of the disease lice must be common, and they are able to infect only one man since the louse must be killed in order to spread the disease. Relapsing fever is also carried by mites, ticks and bed-bugs.

## Crab Lice

There can be few personal discoveries more disconcerting than to find that one is infested by the crab louse, *Phthirus pubis*. They were described by Linnaeus in 1758, but now they are far more common than body lice and their increase in numbers has been likened to an epidemic. There are probably several hundred thousand people infested in Britain. In the past crabs were associated with prostitutes and the lower deck, but many a self-esteeming lady has recently gone to the surgery reduced to speechlessness and finger-pointing.

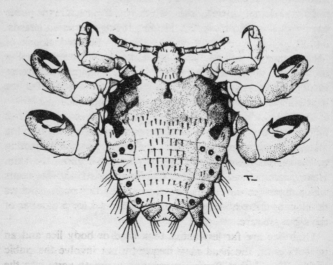

*Crab louse*

As their French name, *papillon d'amour*, implies, they are almost always acquired through sexual intercourse. They are sedentary in their habits and require close contact to be exchanged, but they can also be transferred on towels and an occasional infestation has been traced to picking up hairs with lice or nits attached from the proverbial lavatory seat. One doctor described to me how he had combed a large number from the pubic hair of a female patient and had deliberately let them drop on the carpet where they crawled about for half an hour, and were clearly in a fit state to colonize somebody else. They bear a striking resemblance to crabs with an abdomen broader than it is long and are easily distinguished from head or body lice. The front pair of legs are much more slender than the second and third which are equipped with strong, curved claws adapted to grasp hairs. The crab louse prefers to clasp coarse hair, and this determines its habitat. For the same reason it is seldom found on children before puberty.

Its main headquarters, as its Latin name implies, are the pubic hairs, but it is also frequently found under the arms, in beards, eyelashes and sometimes on the sparsely forested slopes of balding pates. The population of adult lice on an individual is usually less than ten as an infestation normally causes intense itching after several weeks of feeding, but as many as 100 lice have been found on the eyelashes of a single individual.

The louse is so well camouflaged and so small (1–2 millimetres long) that it is hard to find even with a magnifying glass, but after feeding they swell and become deep red, ejecting pellets of reddish excrement which are strewn about the skin. Heavy infestations also produce characteristic bluish spots which appear in the deeper tissues caused by tiny haemorrhages developing some hours after a bite. These last for a number of days, but are rare.

Crab lice are far less active than head or body lice and an infestation on the head may frequently not involve the pubic region. They travel slowly, inserting their mouth-parts into the skin and feeding intermittently as many as twelve times a day, but it is thought that the females tend — on hairy individuals —

to move away from the pubic regions onto the trunk to lay their eggs. So it is ineffective to treat only the pubic region with insecticides.

The complete life cycle takes about twenty-five days. The eggs are cemented to hairs next to the skin, and are laid at the rate of about five a day up to a total of twenty-six. They hatch in a week and then pass through three larval stages in thirteen to seventeen days. The adult lives for about a month, but being dependent on the blood of the human host it will die within twenty-four hours if separated. Infestations frequently run in families and can be passed from mothers to the scalp and eyelashes of infants. Crab lice appear to dislike the close-growing hair of adults' and children's scalps.

Social attitudes to the crab louse prevent many infested individuals from getting proper treatment and ineffective attempts at self-medication with agents as different and painful as petrol, fly spray, and dog-flea powders are common. One classic naval 'cure' used to be rum and sand, both easily procurable on board ship, and applied on the basis that the lice would get raging drunk and stone each other to death!

On one occasion John Maunder of the London School of Hygiene and Tropical Medicine received a letter from a student at Stirling University expressing no confidence in the Student Health Service and complaining of a local epidemic of crabs; at the same time the Service wrote asking for advice on the best treatment. Maunder inserted a coupon in the University paper offering confidential advice — and did not get a single reply. He now believes that crab lice are a frequent cause of people's failure to go to VD treatment centres — they are too embarrassed.

Considering its close association with man, remarkably little is known about the crab louse, one problem being that until recently it was not possible to feed them successfully on artificial media. Volunteers who wear them strapped to their arms in bottomless boxes become sensitized after a while and cannot tolerate them. In the meantime the suspicion has been aroused that although they do not carry typhus they can transmit syphilis.

There are only two men studying lice in Britain, Maunder and Burgess, indeed they are, to my knowledge, the only scientists working on head and crab lice in the whole world. Considering how many of us are infested and how our health can suffer from their attentions this would seem, without beating about the bush, to be stupidly shortsighted.

## 9
# Bed Bugs

*He had scraped together a handful of bugs from the bed-clothes and crushed them under a candle-stick, and had done that many a time when he had to resort to the lowest places.*

MAYHEW, *London Labour and the London Poor*

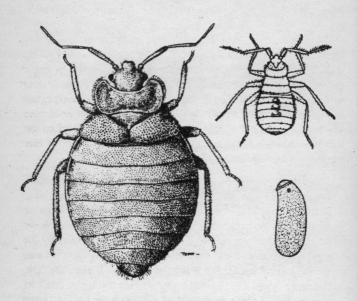

*Bed bug.* Left, *adult male;* right, *egg and newly hatched nymph (Drawings not to same scale)*

The bed bug, compared with the louse, has a very different form of parasitic association with man. It lives in cracks in walls or furniture, or in the seams of mattresses, where it also lays its eggs, and it can feed on other warm-blooded animals as well as man. It also has a much longer lifespan and is able to survive as an adult for as long as a year and a half, so that a single bug can be an irritating pest over a long period.

Coming as they do in the dead of night to steal their drops of blood from a sleeper's throat or face like diminutive vampires, bugs are held in a very special dread. If a house is infested no amount of slaughter will stop others from creeping up the moment sleep sets in, and it is almost as bad to have a single crafty bug which waits with predatory intent for the moment when exhaustion causes sleep to take over from nervous watchfulness.

In former times their presence was accepted as one of the hazards of town life, and a brisk sale was made of cures. During the eighteenth and nineteenth centuries there was a business carried on by three generations of the Tiffin family in the Strand in London. The grandfather had been a ladies' stay-maker, but the father would go about his work in the houses of noblemen and carriage company, complete with powdered wig, cocked hat and sword, while the son styled himself 'Bug destroyer to Her Majesty'. Mayhew quotes him:

> I was once at work on the Princess Charlotte's own bedstead. I was in the room and she asked me if I had found anything, and I told her no; but just at that minute I did happen to catch one, and upon that she sprang upon the bed, and put her hand on my shoulder to look at it. She had been tormented by the creature, because I was ordered to come directly and that was the only one I found. When the Princess saw it, she said, 'Oh, the nasty thing! That's what tormented me last night; don't let him escape.' I think he looked all the better for having tasted Royal blood.

The poor were reduced to drinking alcohol to lower their sensitivity to the bites.

Bed bugs are divided by climate. *Cimex lectularius* pesters white men in temperate zones and *Cimex hemipterus* those with black skins in the tropics. They belong to the order Heteroptera, a large group of insects which have piercing and sucking mouth-parts. Nearly all of the group use their mouth-parts to suck the juices of plants, and many are agricultural pests. It is likely that the bed bug's ancestors were parasites of birds and bats which transferred their attentions to man when he began to live in caves and stayed with their new host when he moved away from the forests into other living quarters.

*C. lectularius* probably originated in a warm climatic area such as the Middle East. Certainly the bed bug did not reach England until the sixteenth century, an unwelcome accompaniment to increasing maritime trade. Mouffet records that

> in the year 1503 Dr Penny was called in great haste to a little village called Mortlake [*now a suburb of London*], near the Thames, to visit two noblemen who were much frightened by the appearance of bug-bites, and were in fear of I know not what contagion; but when the matter was known, and the insects caught, he laughed them out of all fear.

Mayhew states that the original name was Chinche or wall-louse and that the name 'bug' had a Welsh origin signifying a ghost or goblin as in the English 'bugbear'. He goes on: 'Hence the passage in the Psalms "thou shalt not be afraid for the terror by night," is rendered in Matthew's bible, "thou shalt not nede to be afraid of any bugs by night." ' To modern ears this falls a bit flat.

Certainly the bed bug has been present in the Mediterranean since classical times. According to Greek legend, when Bacchus went down into Hell he pleaded with Jupiter that the inns on the return journey should be bug-free. The Romans called the bed bug *Cimex,* and swallowed it washed down with water or wine as a cure for complaints varying from strangulation to snake-bite, but when Linnaeus later adopted the Latin name he was under the impression that the bug was not a native of Europe and had been imported from America.

Bed bugs are still far more common in non-industrial countries than is usually appreciated. My sister-in-law described to me how, as a child in Eastern Turkey, they had always put bean-leaves upside-down in a ring around the legs of young children's beds. In the morning they would find bugs trapped on the hairs of the leaves and would drop them in the river.

In Britain bed bugs seem a thing of the past, but as recently as 1934 one house in ten was infested in major cities. School-teachers in the poorer parts of London would describe how children would sleep on the doorsteps in summer to avoid the insects, and how the yawning child rubbing its eyes would be the result (in those days before television) of a bug-ridden home. Even when slums were cleared the bugs would be carried with the furniture to the new housing estates, and because of the association with dirty living conditions an area reputed to have bugs was soon shunned by cleaner families, so bed bugs were even credited with creating slums rather than just being a part of them. But within ten years the incidence had fallen to one house infested in 100 and by 1963 it had fallen to one in 10 000. Disinfestation squads still operate, spraying rooms with BHC dissolved in paraffin (to the horror of the fire-brigade), and there is no doubt that DDT has been instrumental in removing this curse from modern life. Even in the tropics the malaria-control DDT spraying has reduced the bug population, except where they are already becoming resistant. But in Britain the first BHC-resistant bug has already been found, and the bug population is growing in high-rise flats in Glasgow where it finds a secure refuge in the ducting leading from flat to flat. I have little doubt that the bed bug is starting to make a comeback.

Most blood-sucking insects are associated with the transmission of disease, and it was somewhat surprising that until recently no one had blamed the bed-bug. But a 1977 review in *Nature* shows that they can be vectors for hepatitis B virus, especially in West Africa. Since we still have no medicines to cure virus diseases, hepatitis can be dangerous.

The adult bed bug is about 6 millimetres long, mahogany-brown and oval, with vestiges of wings like two scales on its back. Its flat profile enables it to scuttle into cracks with surprising speed. It has long antennae and its eyes probably do no more than enable it to distinguish light from dark and the outline of menacing shadows. Very little is known about the methods a bed bug uses to track down its host. It has been claimed that even if a bed is stood with its legs in bowls of water the bug will still seek out its victim by dropping off the ceiling, but the story is apocryphal. However, it can wait for a long time for a meal, up to 500 days if the temperature is low. Bed bugs will feed about every sixth day at 15°C but every night at 25°C. As is normal with insects their rate of metabolism is regulated by temperature, but they can survive several months at freezing point.

Bed bugs usually live in cracks speckled with faeces in the bed frame itself or in the wall close to a bed, but there are well-authenticated cases where bugs will migrate from one bedroom to another. The bed bug is also equipped with a large gland under the thorax which emits a characteristic stink when the insect is disturbed and a sensitive nose will discern an infested house.

It carries its proboscis folded backwards under its head and during feeding, which takes five to ten minutes, two outer pairs of stylets lance the skin with rows of teeth while an inner pair are pressed together to form a tube up which the blood is drawn. An unfed bug is quite flat, but the body is distended and elongated by the meal which can be seen as a purple colour through the cuticle of the young insect. The peak time for feeding is between 3.00 a.m. and 6.00 a.m., and a light left burning will deter bugs to some extent. Eggs are laid at the rate of about three a day and are glued to the sides of the crack where the female lives. The more often she feeds, the more she lays and the eggs total about 100 if the bug is well fed. Like hens they also lay infertile eggs if they have not been fertilized by one or more males. The fertile eggs hatch after about three weeks and there are five nymphal stages each resembling diminutive adults. The whole reproductive cycle is completed after about three months. The egg shells usually remain attached to the laying place but sometimes the larvae can be seen moving about like young partridges with the shells stuck to their backs.

At present in Britain infestations are only common in animal houses where they can be a troublesome source of bacterial cross-infection to laboratory animals. But people unfortunate enough to be bitten react in markedly different ways. Professor J. B. S. Haldane once startled a Royal Society conversazione by demonstrating publicly that he was immune to their bites. Some people show no sign of a bite at all, while others will swell up with large blisters like the most violent reaction to a nettle sting. This can often lead to confusion as to which rooms in a house are infested.

But even bed bugs have their uses. A few years ago *Time* magazine published a photograph of a US Marine carrying what was called a 'people sniffer', a tubular device with horn-like pipes pointing forwards. The accompanying article explained that it worked on the principle that when a bed bug scents man it stamps around eagerly and the amplified patter of tiny feet could be used as a warning of approaching Viet Cong. When I inquired for more details the US Marines denied all knowledge of the device. Either it was on the secret list or the bugs must have shown a predilection for American blood.

# 10
# Learning to Live with our Ecology

*We are quietly and innocently killing lots of patients.*
A bacteriologist in 1975

Ecology is a fashionable and much-abused word, but the day when American astronauts first pointed a television camera at the Earth from space was not the first time man had realized that he was dependent on his surroundings. No farmer who has scanned the skies in search of rain would consider himself independent of the great cycles of drought and plenty which Nature bestows. But man does not treat his environment rationally; if Rachel Carson and her book, *Silent Spring,* awoke us to the dangers of the indiscriminate use of pesticides, it has not stopped the housewife seizing a fly-spray to contaminate otherwise clean food, and appallingly toxic compounds are bought with enthusiasm in every gardening shop. A sense of proportion between contamination by flies or DDT can be based only on a knowledge of the facts. If nurses remain unaware that lice are bloodsucking insects, and if doctors have no understanding of the ecological effects of their drugs, we are likely to get into a worse mess than we are already. We must also learn to think in terms of the interactions of the flora and fauna of our skins, which affect not only ourselves but others. It is not just a question of picking up and bestowing fleas, we share our micro-organisms too.

Every movement we make, every flexing of our skin is accompanied by a tiny shower of skin particles released into the air. About 10 000 million skin scales or squames peel off each of our bodies every twenty-four hours. Seen through the microscope even the finest nylon stocking looks like wire netting which acts like a cheese-grater on the outer layers of the epidermis. At first static electricity holds the tiny flakes to the mesh of material, then they float free into the air.

We are well aware of these particles, they are the motes in the sunbeam stretched across a darkened room. House dust consists of 80–90 per cent skin, and each of us sheds from one to one-and-a-half grams of skin a day, about one pound every year. That grey dust that settles on the top of your wardrobe and fills your vacuum-cleaner is 90 per cent skin. If you doubt it, try burning some and the characteristic smell of burning keratin, the same as from burning hair or when a blacksmith puts a hot shoe against a horse's hoof, will confirm it.

It is thought that most skin is shed when we are in bed or undressing as it is then that there is most friction against the skin, and measurements made on volunteers in a series of highly peculiar scientific experiments confirm that there is little shedding from the trunk compared with the limbs. The experiments were done to determine the amount of skin shed and also to discover to what extent skin scales were contaminated with bacteria. They began by washing a scientist's socks.

After a day's wear the socks were washed out in sterile solution so that the skin scales could be separated, dried and weighed. The average pair of socks traps about 190 milligrams of skin a day, but a vest only a quarter of that amount, although such thick material as wool traps most of the skin shed. Stocking tights, however, trapped less skin than a pair of socks in spite of the far greater skin area covered, and so it was revealed that the mini-skirt had an anti-social effect undreamed of by admirers of the female form.

Next to the skin is a thin layer of air which is warmed by the body. Because it is warmed it flows upwards, and a naked man or woman standing erect is enveloped in a moving current of air 1 or 2 centimetres thick over the lower legs and 20 centimetres thick at the face, where it will be moving upwards at a speed of about 30 centimetres a second.

Skin particles released through clothing are caught up in this boundary-layer flow, which exists even outside a person's clothes, and are whisked upwards into the surrounding air. A girl in a mini-skirt will scatter about 300 milligrams of skin scales a day while a man wearing thick trousers will probably only release his skin scales when he undresses in the bedroom. The point is that skin scales are densely populated with microorganisms. A bacterial count on a staircase showed 750 organisms per cubic metre of air, but after brushing the stairs for ten minutes the count went up to 410 000.

About 330 skin scales settle on 1 square millimetre of a laboratory bench top (or a food counter or a hospital floor) every day, a gently falling snow of skin laden with germs; and if a person sneezed continuously he would still produce only a tenth of the number of particles that are shed from his skin, so it becomes very important just what the organisms on our skin are. Every single skin scale examined in the laboratory was found to be contaminated and two-thirds of them carried large colonies of bacteria. Whether these colonies survive depends on the weather; left in humid air the colonies would grow on their skin rafts alone. The survival of bacteria on their little rafts of skin varies from species to species. Staphylococci and micrococci resist drying better than diphtheroids, while the fungus *Candida* is killed by drying out.

Although most bacteria on the skin surface are commensals which are harmless, large areas of our bodies are frequently contaminated with potentially dangerous pathogenic organisms; these could obviously be a source of infection when breathed in. It could be that fresh air fiends who believe in leaving all the windows open might indeed be reducing the numbers of contaminated particles in their immediate environment.

It has also just been discovered that viruses can travel in skin scales, and it is possible that they are incorporated into the cell as it grows in the epidermis. Many virus diseases such as measles and German measles go through a stage when the virus is present in large quantities in the blood reaching the skin through the capillaries or from inflamed areas forming a rash. If it is true that the virus can localize in the skin, after several weeks an individual who has had the disease may be shedding large quantities of virus into the air in his skin scales. At the Medical Research Council Laboratory, Holly Hill, Hampstead, polio virus has already been demonstrated to exist on shed skin, but nobody as yet knows for certain if it got there from the bloodstream. Until more work is done it is impossible to say how serious this mode of infection is.

In the ordinary way the resident populations on our skins and the cilia (sweeping bristles) in our air passages protect us from the incursions of foreign organisms, but there is one place where our tissues lie open to immediate attack — in the operating theatre. Particularly prone to infection are patients who undergo long operations such as the replacement of hip joints. And the most dangerous of our micro-organisms to them are the so-called opportunist bacteria which will flourish in a wound. The most important of these is *Staphylococcus aureus*. Patients have even been found to be infecting themselves with their own bacteria, but the main concern in hospitals is the risk of cross-infection by resistant organisms.

Early research on bacterial populations showed that one person in every ten is likely to disperse large quantities of *Staphylococcus aureus* and that operating theatre personnel were as likely as any others to be dispersers. The first reaction was that all would be well if the surgeon and nurses had a shower before operating, extending the scrubbing-up treatment to the whole body. But then to the dismay of the bacteriologists who made samples of bacteria released into the air it was found that after a shower a person would release two and a half times as many bacteria into the air as one who had not showered, because the large colonies on the skin were broken up and more easily dispersed. It was then found that the bacterial counts were almost as bad whether they were naked or had surgical gowns on. Measurements showed that more than a million viable bacteria could be shed by a person spending forty minutes in a sterile room.

Clearly if the patient could be isolated from the team by

enclosing him in a plastic capsule with his own air supply contamination from skin scales could be eliminated, and several different techniques of this kind have been developed including some in which the surgeon works in a plastic suit. But anything which reduces the surgeon's skill by hampering his movement or tiring him during a long operation is counter-productive. So experiments were done to find out which part of the body shed most bacteria.

Even by enclosing the ends of sleeves and trouser-legs bacterial contamination of the air could be reduced ten-fold, and suits of closely woven material halved the numbers again. Other research showed that the most important area for shedding was the groin, so it is likely that before long it will become common practice for operating theatre staff to be equipped with closely woven skin-scale-proof underpants. Ironically it was found that compared with the contamination from skin scales, hardly any bacteria were breathed out. Evidently the surgical mask might be better employed covering different orifices of the body.

It has been traditional for surgeons to 'scrub-up' their hands before an operation, and this was encouraged by research which claimed that it was possible completely to disinfect the skin. But in 1972 Sydney Selwyn of the Westminster Hospital published results which demonstrated unequivocally that at least 20 per cent of the bacteria resident on the skin were impervious to the most rigorous cleaning even with iodine, because either they lie deep in the hair follicles or sebaceous glands, or in skin crevices between protecting layers of keratinized cells. Far from being a problem, it is extremely fortunate that this is so because the remaining bacteria are not only harmless, they positively aid the skin in defending itself against invading opportunist organisms such as *Staphylococcus aureus*.

Scrubbing-up does however remove the transient bacteria which contaminate our skins from other sources, but these are relatively easily removed. As Dr Selwyn says: 'Surgeons' hands are delicate instruments and there is no need to treat them as if they were floors.'

Attitudes to antisepsis have changed greatly since the

discovery of the antibiotics. When Joseph Lister in 1867 began to use carbolic disinfectant to prevent bacteria reaching wounds during operation he revolutionized a situation where 'surgical fever' caused by infection was so common that a contemporary colleague had said 'Every patient placed upon an operation table is in greater danger than a soldier entering one of the bloodiest and most fatal battlefields.'

Before he used carbolic, fatalities after amputations were as high as 43 per cent of all cases; afterwards the figure dropped to 15 per cent, a mortality rate that would be totally unacceptable today. Yet 10 per cent of operation wounds still become infected. The complexity and length of operations carried out today would astound Lister, yet the principle of excluding bacteria from the wound is just as vital, but there is still no routine sampling of air contamination in British operating theatres. The theory of airborne contamination is well known but lack of money, shortage of staff and human inertia have so far stopped any application on behalf of the patient.

Just how serious the situation can be was shown in 1963 at St Albans City Hospital. An anaesthetist had been found to be a carrier of *Staphylococcus aureus* three years previously at another hospital, and he had been off work with psoriasis, a skin disease which leads to excessive scaling of the skin. After his condition was treated with steroids it cleared up and he returned to work. Within two weeks there were thirty-three operating theatre infections reported which resulted in four deaths. These were traced to airborne contamination by bacteria from the anaesthetist. This was an extreme case, but mild cases of skin infection caused by dangerous *Staphylococci* are common. These may not even be visible to the naked eye and are a major source of infection.

It is ironic that Florence Nightingale who did so much to humanize and regulate the treatment of patients in hospital should steadfastly have refused to believe in bacteria, and patients still die as the result of her views. At the Aberdeen Royal Infirmary the surgical ward was built on the Nightingale plan, as in the majority of hospitals, with beds lined down the walls of a large open ward. It was then converted to compartments and single rooms with the result that post-operative wound infection dropped from 14.5 per cent to 7 per cent. There was a hundred-fold reduction in Staphylococcal particle counts, and an epidemic strain of resistant *Staphylococcus* disappeared.

Infection in hospital is a vast subject on its own, and is probably the cause of the deep-seated mistrust of hospital shared by many of the older generation who can remember too vividly the days when Streptococcal infections like puerperal fever (child-bed fever) and scarlet fever were all too commonly fatal. The *Streptococci* are still sensitive to penicillin and often still to tetracycline and it is now *Staphylococcus aureus*, the gram negative bacilli and the formidable virus of serum hepatitis which are most to be feared. It is now widely recognized that after an operation the shortest possible stay in hospital is the best.

Infection can be spread by such widely differing objects as stethoscopes, ants, beards, hands, humidifiers, and even supposedly antiseptic solutions. And the control of hospital micro-organisms has at last begun to be treated on an ecological basis. For a long time it had been current practice to wash down hospital floors and equipment with hexachlorophene which kills gram positive bacteria such as *Staphylococci*. Unfortunately, it was ineffective against some gram negative organisms including the bacillus *Pseudomonas aeruginosa* which is an extremely important source of infection in large wounds and especially burns. These bacteria are found in every hospital, and being adapted to moist conditions, they flourish in places such as vases of flowers, sink plugs, hospital baths and shaving brushes. It was found by Professor Harvey Blank, Professor of Dermatology in an American hospital, that the extensive use of hexachlorophene allowed the invasion of *Pseudomonas* more than when detergents only or broad-spectrum antiseptics were used. Fortunately concentrations of the bacteria fluoresce under ultra-violet radiation, and routine checks with ultra-violet light were begun which showed up not only colonies on equipment but also the infected areas of wounds. The programme was so successful in reducing post-operative infection that the surgeons invited the dermatology department to share the running of their ward, an almost unheard-of delegation of responsibility!

The control of potentially harmful organisms which arrive on our bodies is not solely due to the pressure of numbers of an existing established population. The task of keeping the skin free from contamination in the anal area would seem almost impossible bearing in mind the wide bacterial flora of the intestine, yet within an hour or so of smearing with faeces the skin supports only its resident *Staphylococci* and diphtheroids. I have mentioned in Chapter 4 the importance of dryness and sebum, but there is another type of interaction between the bacteria themselves which is undoubtedly a help to our immunity.

In 1972 Dr Selwyn showed that there were strains of bacteria present on about one in every five individuals which actively inhibited the growth of resistant *Staphylococcus aureus* by the production of their own antibiotics. He isolated thirty-two different strains of Micrococcaceae with this capacity and went on to show that patients equipped with these strains on their skins had a fifth or less chance of becoming infected during surgery than those without them. What is more, the patients with the defending organisms who were infected were colonized by different organisms, gram negative rather than gram positive bacteria.

If these defending organisms are so effective it seems puzzling that only one in five of us should be colonized by them. The likely reason is that they have no specific advantage on normal skin and perhaps are even a disadvantage. It is only in the moist environment of a wound that natural selection favours their multiplication at the expense of other species.

Faced with the increasing resistance of Staphylococcal strains to artificial antibiotics, this discovery would seem to be a timely opportunity to set bacteria to catch bacteria in the same way that biological methods have been used to control pests with their own predators. At present Dr Selwyn has a research project under way on animals. As he says, he would love to be able to inoculate patients with the defending bacteria as they walked in the hospital door, 'but we are in an age when people are rightly cautious and we need more knowledge before letting them loose on our patients.'

Dermatological magazines, with their weird juxtaposition of advertisements displaying supple slinky nudes and photographs of grotesque clinical deformities are now carrying more and more articles on the interactions of our skin flora. One condition currently in great dispute and where there are rich pickings for the private consultant is acne.

Diseases are not the subject of this book, but the striking thing about acne is that it may be caused by the action of one of our normal skin bacteria, and it is so common amongst teenagers that it can almost be considered normal. It is an affliction peculiar to the human species.

One study in Boston, Mass. showed that 77–99 per cent of the fourteen-to-eighteen-year-old age-group suffered from acne, but the girls had milder attacks than boys. It is by far the most common skin disorder and normally appears when the concentration of male hormones increases in the bloodstream leading to an increase in the size and activity of the sebaceous glands. It usually first appears on the nose of adolescents spreading outwards to the cheek and beard area. There are also cases where girls who have been taking the contraceptive Pill find that they get oily skins a month after stopping the Pill and that acne follows a couple of months later. These attacks can last about six months but are not severe and seldom result in the scarring which bad cases of acne cause.

In the normal sebaceous follicle the skin scales are shed and are carried out of the follicle in a continuous stream. The events that lead up to acne begin with these skin scales sticking together to form a dense plug or comedo, known as a blackhead as the reaction with air and the melanin particles in the skin give it a dark colour. This prevents the further flow of sebum to the skin and the anaerobic diphtheroid *Corynebacterium acnes* then sets to work. This is a normal member of our skin flora which is present in numbers of at least 100 000 to the square centimetre in abundant sebaceous follicles. The bacteria split down the secretions of sebum into free fatty acids which begin to attack the wall of the follicle which then bursts, allowing the bacteria to come in contact with the tissue of the epidermis causing red inflamed spots or papules. White cells are mobilized to attack the bacteria and form pus which in turn forms pustules.

The result is sufficiently unpleasant to make 90 per cent of those who suffer resort to some form of self-medication and Americans spend over £30 million a year on doubtful therapy. The affliction tends to recede in spring and summer and appears to be self-limiting in that once a follicle has been infected it will not succumb again. No one knows why stress such as exams may cause a sudden flare-up of spots.

Treatment had been to increase the scaling of the surface skin scales either by making the skin cells proliferate more quickly with vitamin A acid cream, or by peeling the skin with substances like sulphur, resorcinol, salicylic acid and benzoyl peroxide. In severe cases tetracyclines are used which markedly reduce the number of *C. acnes*. At lower doses it appears that tetracyclines interfere with the splitting of sebum into fatty acids, again improving the condition.

Nevertheless the spots are often extremely resistant to treatment, and it is perhaps for this reason that they have been linked with teenage over-indulgence, particularly with food. That acne has any connection with diet such as chocolate has been disproved by experiment, but diet restriction is a convenient refuge for the harassed doctor who knows of no effective treatment. The encouragement to go on resisting chocolate at least sounds as if it is having a beneficial effect, and if the acne does not clear up momentary relapses of diet can always be blamed!

One American skin specialist became convinced that pressure on sensitive follicles was the cause, noting that the spots appeared where chins are supported on hands, and on lower cheeks which repose on fists, or equally as the result of investigative prodding in front of the mirror. He urged his patients to adopt pattern substitution so that they touched their elbows every time they were going to touch the sensitive area, and claimed a high rate of success.

That acne should come just when young people are most conscious of their appearance is one of the cruel tricks of nature exploited by the fringe pharmaceutical industry. There is very little you can do to stop it other than washing your face with soap and water (which will also keep down the follicle mite which is thought to be a complicating factor in some cases). As with baldness there is one sure-fire preventive for the men — eunuchs don't get acne.

Some antibiotics such as tetracyclines when taken by mouth later appear on the skin, and ironically the best test to show that they have reached the skin surface is the presence of bacteria resistant to their action. A typical result is to convert the population of diphtheroid bacteria in the armpits to resistant coccal colonies. In other words administering powerful antibiotics can lead to the possibility of infection by harmful germs in a place not under observation by the doctor, simply because they upset the normal ecological equilibrium. Acne is now often treated with prolonged prescription of tetracyclines. Prolonged use of broad-spectrum antibiotics can result in an overgrowth of yeasts and gram negative bacteria from the bowel.

It is one thing for untoward ecological changes to be caused by drugs given under prescription by a doctor whose training should include an appreciation of the possibility of side-effects, it is a quite different matter if products are on sale to the public which can do the same.

In the last ten years there has been a spectacular boom in the sale of aerosol packaged products, from flysprays and paint to mixtures to stop your hinges squeaking and to make your car start on a damp day. In 1974, 478 million cans were sold in the United Kingdom — eight for every man, woman and child. Consumption was increasing at 15 per cent a year and had a long way to go to catch up the American *per capita* rate which was almost double ours. More than half the aerosol cans sold contained cosmetics, and after hairsprays the next most popular products were antiperspirants and deodorants. Extremely intensive propaganda in women's magazines had pushed the sales of these from eight million cans in 1967 to forty-eight million in 1971. But the manufacturers began to come under heavy criticism on four different counts. First they were accused of creating a demand by making women unnaturally sensitive to natural odours causing anxiety and even psychological disturbance; second, that some of the ingredients which were often secret could be harmful, and third, that they were capable of upsetting the ecological equilibrium of sensitive areas of the body. Fourth, the most commonly used propellants in aerosol sprays are fluoro-carbons which are now suspected to be attacking the upper-atmosphere ozone which shields us from excessive ultra-violet radiation.

Body odour is caused by the action of skin bacteria breaking down the natural secretions from the sebaceous, sweat, and apocrine glands and the simplest and safest way of avoiding it is to wash with soap and water. This, however, was thought by manufacturers to be a sales area ripe for exploitation and there were two ways in which more expensive — and thus more profitable — products could be used. Either the secretions could be discouraged by the simple expedient of blocking up the gland openings with aluminium compounds, the basis of antiperspirants; or the bacterial population could be reduced by antiseptics so that they could not break down the secretions thus reducing undesirable smells.

The disadvantages of over-enthusiastically blocking up sweat glands are obvious, but the effects of removing the normal bacteria are not. Since a large proportion of the deodorants were advertised specifically for 'intimate' or vaginal use (according to their opponents exploiting women's sexual insecurity and the feeling of uncleanliness they may feel when menstruating) they were being used on an area of the body easily contaminated by other organisms and highly susceptible to infection.

The first adverse reports followed the use of under-arm deodorants when it was found that wiping out the normal bacteria allowed invasion of bacteria such as the species proteus from the intestine. These could produce ammonia from normal skin secretions which in turn would cause irritation of the skin. The next stage is for fungi to infect the damaged skin surface which is then frequently misdiagnosed as eczema and treated with cortisone cream which encourages the growth of the fungi leading to a vicious circle of an extreme kind.

By 1972, 74 per cent of women in Britain were using deodorants and 17 per cent were using vaginal deodorants, and skin specialists were having to deal with increasing numbers of cases of extremely distressed women with large inflamed areas of horribly sensitive skin infected by fungi, proteus, and pseudomonas bacteria which had settled in the ecological niche left empty by removing the resident population of bacteria. Once the skin population has been upset in this way it does not always right itself automatically and so far there is no reliable way of restoring the *status quo*. Another problem was that women were using the sprays against medical conditions such as thrush and trichomoniasis which also cause bad smells and which require proper treatment with the right drugs. Whether because of the bad publicity or because of the general tightening of the purse-strings caused by inflation, the number of women using vaginal deodorants fell in the autumn of 1973 to 10 per cent compared with 17 per cent the year before.

In 1973 the United States Food and Drug Administration decided that vaginal deodorants served no useful hygienic purpose and should carry a health warning, but it will take more positive action than that to stop an industry worth £20 million a year in the USA.

A chemical which was widely used in deodorant sprays until 1973 is hexachlorophene. The chemical constituents of cosmetics do not have to be tested for toxicity in the same way that medicines have since the thalidomide tragedy, and it was not until a farmer in Florida applied to use the chemical on his crops as a fungicide that the first animal tests were done. First rats and then monkeys were washed with solutions of hexachlorophene and disquieting evidence appeared that seemed to link the treatment with brain damage. Then in the autumn of 1972 twenty-eight babies died in France, and it was suspected that the cause was a talcum powder which accidentally contained, according to reports, 6 per cent hexachlorophene. Up to 70 per cent of the drug present in the talcum passed through their skins to cause brain damage.

The chemical was then used widely in maternity wards in hospitals to prevent cross-infection. It was dusted on umbilical cords and in many American hospitals babies were washed in it daily. A survey made in two hospitals in Seattle led the investigators to conclude that hexachlorophene was related to brain damage in children. It was not long before the United States Food and Drug Administration decreed that the chemical was only to be sold on a doctor's prescription and banned it from use in soaps and cosmetics. In Britain the Department of Health asked manufacturers to impose a voluntary ban on the use of hexachlorophene in baby preparations and to limit its use in other products to 0.1 per cent. But at present toilet preparations and cosmetics do not have to have their ingredients stated on the package and there is nothing to prevent unscrupulous manufacturers including hexachlorophene. A draft E E C directive is under discussion which will require a limited listing of ingredients, but only a compulsory listing of all ingredients would be an effective deterrent. In the meantime hexachlorophene lotion is still recommended on page 148 of the 1973 New English Library edition of Dr Spock's *Baby and Child Care*. This advice should *not* be followed, as the publishers agreed when I brought the matter to their attention.

While the individual may all too easily damage his micro-flora unwittingly, there are many whose obsessive pre-occupation with cleanliness still cannot remove the natural inhabitants of their skin. While an infestation of lice or scabies causes horror, most people will come to terms with the idea that they are covered with live bacteria; potent as they may be, they don't crawl around on hairy legs.

A horror of insects is a widespread human trait which is not illogical especially in tropical countries where the bites of many are poisonous and some are fatal. But entomologists are frequently plagued themselves by people suffering from a condition they call entomophobia — erroneously believing themselves to be infested with insects. Typical examples are the lady who was quite certain that there were lice inside her crash helmet because every time she rode her motorcycle she could hear them buzzing inside. Perhaps 'bees in her bonnet' derives from the same source. Another man thought that he was the victim of a new kind of louse which was invisible but hung from strings all over his house at exactly the right height to bite him on the nose.

These are cases for the psychiatrist, but doctors should beware of confusing them with the infestations I have mentioned in the chapter on mites.

When the Apollo 12 mission touched down on the Moon in 1971 astronauts recovered a camera which had spent two years on the Moon's surface. When it was taken back to Houston the scientists who examined it found that it was still contaminated with bacteria from the earth that had survived the journey to the Moon and two years in the vacuum of space.

Wherever man goes he is not alone. Though we may leave the Earth we take with us on any voyage of discovery our own personal world which is yet to be completely explored. We evolved on Earth, but we did so in the company of the minute creatures which live out their lives on our bodies.

We should treat our fellow travellers with respect; they are much more adaptable than we are, and they do us more good than harm.

# Bibliography

J. R. Busvine, *Insects and Hygiene* Methuen 1966.

J. R. Busvine, *Insects, Hygiene and History* Athlone Press 1977.

C. Creighton, *A History of Epidemics in Britain from A.D. 664 to the Extinction of Plague* Cambridge University Press 1891.

B. Dixon, *Invisible Allies: Microbes and Man's Fate* Maurice Temple Smith, 1976.

C. Dobell (editor), *Antony Van Leeuwenhoek and his 'Little Animals'* Dover Publications Inc. 1960.

H. I. Maibach (editor), *Skin Bacteria and their Rôle in Infection* McGraw Hill 1965.

M. J. Marples, *The Ecology of the Human Skin* C. C. Thomas 1965.

K. Mellanby, *Human Guinea Pigs* Merlin Press 1973.

T. Rosebury, *Microorganisms Indigenous to Man* McGraw Hill 1962.

M. Rothschild and T. Clay, *Fleas, Flukes and Cuckoos* Collins 1952.

K. G. V. Smith (editor), *Insects and other Arthropods of Medical Importance* British Museum (Natural History) 1973.

H. Zinser, *Rats, Lice, and History* George Routledge and Sons Ltd. 1935.

# Acknowledgements

Since this book is written for a non-specialist public it contains no footnotes or references. However, it could not have been written without the help of a large number of books, articles, letters and interviews. I owe a debt to the scientific community at large, and particularly to the following:

J. Almeida, W. G. Barnes, H. Blank, R. Blowers, W. D. Brighton, J. R. Busvine, R. P. Clark, T. O. Coston, F. P. English, R. R. Gillies, D. A. Griffiths, J. Lees, M. J. Marples, R. R. Marples, J. Maunder, K. Mellanby, The Hon. Miriam Rothschild, S. Selwyn, F. G. A. M. Smith, K. G. V. Smith, J. A. Swift, M. G. R. Varma.

# Index